BIRTH OF A FAMILY

Nathan Cabot Hale

BIRTH OF
A FAMILY

The New Role of the Father in Childbirth

FOREWORD BY JESSICA DICK-READ

ANCHOR BOOKS
Anchor Press/Doubleday, Garden City, New York
1979

The Anchor Books edition is the first publication of *Birth of a Family*.

Anchor Books edition: 1979

Library of Congress Cataloging in Publication Data

Hale, Nathan Cabot.
 Birth of a family.

 1. Natural childbirth. 2. Fathers. I. Title.
RG661.H34   616.4'5'024041
ISBN: 0-385-14162-9
Library of Congress Catalog Card Number 78–68340

This book is dedicated to the memory of Grantly Dick-Read, M.D., and to those men who are in the process of becoming fathers. It is my hope that they will find herein thoughts of value which will advance the heritage, lore, and art of fatherhood.

FOREWORD

It was the smile of a newborn babe that inspired the author to write this book and, in the face of ignorance, arrogance, and the materialistic concepts of a certain junta of the world's medical profession, he has, with strengthened determination and courage, passed on through the eyes of a layman his personal observations, in writing and pictorial fact, of the truth and beauty of natural childbirth.

It is classically self-explanatory and its appeal should touch the hearts of all true men to whom it is dedicated.

Other than to remember the smile of that newborn, this very lovely book needs no influential backing, for it will receive its acclaim on merit alone. But I do believe it is now up to Man to meet the challenge to accord him his rightful place as a respective Father-to-be and, together with his partner, enforce that right's being recognized and ensured.

There should also be no place for discord between doctors and their patients, for mutual understanding lays no claim to barriers.

JESSICA DICK-READ

ACKNOWLEDGMENTS

For making it possible for me to observe the miracle of birth, for friendship and brotherhood:

John W. Grover, M.D.

For encouragement, help, and advice:

Marie Dutton Brown
Margie Chiumento
Jessica Dick-Read
Mary Gruskin
Alison B. Hale
Arthur Nelson, M.D.

My special gratitude is also owed to a great and progressive medical institution:

The Boston Hospital for Women
A Division of the Affiliated Hospitals Center, Inc.
221 Longwood Avenue
Boston, Massachusetts 02115

THE ROLE OF THE FATHER IN CHILDBIRTH

This is a book about childbirth from the father's point of view. It has been written by a man for men. It is not a medical textbook and has not been written by a medical doctor. It is a book written about things that are common to all ordinary men in the process of childbirth. It is a book about the seldom respected, sadly neglected instinct of fatherhood.

There are those who deny that there is any such instinct, but what is written here is intended to help men find that instinct. The fact is that science hasn't learned very much yet about the instincts that we men have about fathering. Until now, medical science has concentrated on the reproductive process of the female organism, on the emotions of motherhood, on the embryo, and on the infant, but aside from the purely physiological aspects of male participation in procreation, there has been no great understanding of the fathering process.

This has really been a matter of scientific firsts, and any sensible man will agree that it is of first importance that women come through childbirth safely and that newborn children are healthy and sound. But now that science can assure these things, it is time for us to explore our own instincts, capacities, and needs in the process of childbirth and the formation of our families. This is particularly important at this time because for the first time in history the family itself is seriously threatened and its future in question.

Of all of the human instincts, the instincts of fatherhood are less understood and more taken for granted by Western culture than any of the other human qualities. Women and youth, in recent times, have made serious attempts at self-questioning and consciousness-raising, and I believe that men will also have to experience a period of self-examination and soul-searching in order for us to find our place and fulfill our responsibilities in the new era of childbirth that we are entering. Since we don't yet know very much at all about the instincts of fathering, this is more of a *why-to* book than a *how-to* book. I will discuss general feelings and possible ways of participating more fully in childbirth, leaving really technical matters of labor and childbirth to the books and classes that deal exclusively in those areas.

What I *will* be doing in this book is to share the impressions, questions, and general concepts about fathering that I have gained through years of study, self-examination, and observation of human emotion, movement, and relationships as a sculptor of the human family and as a scientist working in the field of morphology. Although I *won't* be giving you all the answers, I will be giving you a *feeling for* the kind of problems that you will encounter in trying to help your wife through labor and childbirth. I believe that, by sharing my experiences and insights with you, I can help you find solutions to your own unique problems as you encounter them in the creation of your family. I am not being modest in saying I don't have all the answers. It is just that I have learned that the most important aspects of the father's relationship to labor and childbirth are unique, having to do with the kind of person he is, the kind of person his wife is, and their ability to work together as a team.

In the text that is to follow, I will discuss a specific method of natural childbirth that is the most gentle for the infant and rewarding for the mother and father. This technique was invented by Dr. Frederick Leboyer and is described in his book *Birth Without Violence.* I will also discuss some of the natural childbirth methods that help the woman in labor and enable the father to participate by helping her through the pains of the labor contractions. My comments are based on my observations of childbirth made with patients of Dr. John W. Grover of Boston, one of this country's foremost practitioners of the Leboyer method. Dr. Grover's patients allowed me to photograph them at home, during labor, and in the delivery room, and to share with them the experience of birth. In doing this, I experienced a genuine rebirth of my own that, among other things, has brought forth this book.

Out of respect for the scientific responsibilities of my friend Dr. Grover, and the many sensitive and caring physicians like him, I want to stress the fact that I am not giving medical advice, I am dealing with the *premedical functions* and feelings of fatherhood: the feelings of male responsibility, love, concern, and protectiveness for wife and children. I am encouraging the growth of an intelligent lore of fatherhood among men in a man-to-man talk. I am also encouraging you and your wife to find physicians like Dr. Grover, who will medically support your natural feelings and help you to participate as fully as you can in the birth of your family.

In the following pages we will discuss "myths of childbirth" that have held back the participation of fathers in childbirth; scientific developments that have begun to dispel these old myths; new ways that fathers can participate in the birth of their families; and the experiences with the Leboyer delivery process of four young couples. At the end of the book, I have listed three favorite books of mine for future study for your preparation in founding your new family.

The Myth of the Disinterested Father

"I heard my wife screaming in the labor room and they wouldn't let me go to her." That statement was made to me by a friend of many years, a man who fought through the Battle of the Bulge, had toughed-out six months in a German prison camp, a man who is master of his trade, a man who has raised three bright and talented children. His wife is every bit as fine, bright, and talented as he is, and if you talk to her, she won't leave any doubt in your mind that she needed her man with her when she was having all of her babies and particularly during that first frightening time. But in those days husbands were not generally allowed to be with their wives in labor or to witness the birth of their children, even if they consciously wanted to. Men were automatically excluded from experiencing the miracle of birth with their wives, regardless of their proven courage, intelligence, or emotional needs.

Why have men been excluded from the birth process? Was there ever any valid reason for this? It was often said that it was *unnatural* for a man to want to be with his wife at this time because it was a purely female affair. It was also implied that any interest in the process of childbirth was not very masculine. But were there ever any sound medical and scientific reasons why the father should have been kept out of the labor and delivery rooms? No. . . . there were no sound reasons then, and there are no sound reasons now *except* in instances when there is a medical complication. It is not in the least unnatural or unmanly to want to observe childbirth and to take part in the labor and delivery of one's own children. Curiosity about childbirth and the desire to observe it are about the most basic desires for knowledge that the human being possesses, and in the case of one's own children, the experience may be a deep emotional and biological need. In addition, science is beginning to find that there are many sound reasons why the father *should* share the experiences of labor and delivery with the mother of their child. For one thing, it brings them closer together and forms the strongest of family feelings. A man who loves his woman wants to be with her, to help ease the pain and give her a sense of protection. All that has ever prevented men from doing this are the myths of childbirth.

There are several stock, unflattering caricatures of men in the myths of childbirth. There is the one of the nervous husband who paces up and down the waiting room, smoking countless cigarettes and behaving like an absurd and incompetent fool, who accepts this as his proper place and waits for the doctor to stick his head out of the delivery room door to say "It's a boy" (as though girls were second-class, unwanted citizens!). Another caricature is of the husband who goes to a nearby bar and gets falling-down drunk and misses the whole show because he can't accept the role of sitting passively in the waiting room. And then there is the popular image of the chap who is so totally "masculine" that he has no understanding of women, women's organic functions, childbirth, infants, or any human being under the age of twenty-one. This fellow is portrayed in a way that gives the impression that he is not exactly sure how the woman got pregnant in the first place. But the odd thing about all these caricatures is that they each show real aspects of underlying feelings that men do have about childbirth: 1) Nervousness, concern for the wife, and upset about being excluded from childbirth. 2) The desire to ease the pain, worry, and frustration by *some* available means. 3) The terrible need, which we all have, to show our masculinity at all costs and to hide all of the curiosity that we have of the mysterious, fascinating, and wonderful functions of the female body. This last sort of anxiety is a pretty deep one.

We men have a dreadful concern about doing anything that will make us appear unmanly to other men and to ourselves. This fear may have to do with the way our bodies are constructed because our external sex organs make for a sense of built-in vulnerability and what Freud called "castration anxiety." For this reason, we have to appear tough and ready to defend ourselves. This defensiveness, in one form or another, seems to be a part of all men's characters, and it is a fact that the wound soldiers in combat fear the most is the loss of, or injury to, the genitals. So we all tend to be a mite touchy about our masculinity and sometimes go to great lengths to not show our more kindly and gentle feelings. But in the childbirth situation, we have to learn to not let anxiety rule our lives and choke off our finer emotions. Emotional maturity means that we have the confidence to show our feelings, to be *real men* who are strong and able to be tender, understanding, and gentle to our wives and children.

What men really want to know is how to get along with women; the myth of male disinterest is the farthest thing from the truth. Our greatest happiness in life comes from women, so we should not feel uneasy about learning all that we can about them in order that we may share and assist in the greatest human experience—the creation of a family.

Probably at this point you are thinking that this *sounds* all very well and good, but just how much do *they* want us to know? Isn't it a fact that women really want to keep us out of their secret selves and slightly off balance? My answer to this is No they really don't, underneath it all, but they may have some hang-ups, too, and this brings us to myth number two.

The Myth of Feminine Secrecy

Just as men have a built-in reason for expressing their masculinity, women have built-in organic reasons for the expression of personal shyness, modesty, and defensiveness against the casual and impersonal curiosity of men. The *interior* genitalia of women, their vaginal secretions, and the menstrual cycle have effects on female behavior just as much as the exterior genitalia of men affects ours. Because of their organic sexual functions, women *naturally* require a certain amount of privacy and a more guarded relationship to the world in general. But at the same time, a woman wants and needs to share her innermost self with a beloved man who has demonstrated to her that he cares to know her that deeply. The reason for this is that this kind of sharing by a woman leads toward the creation of a family. Getting to know a woman is a very serious business.

However, just as some men can be extreme about their masculinity, some women also tend to be extreme about their modesty and need to keep men at a distance, to the extent that they have promoted the concept of total feminine secrecy about body functions and childbirth. The mature feminine approach, on the other hand, is the education of boys and men to the understanding of female emotional needs, their reproductive process, and sexual needs.

The simple truth is that men who are educated about women's functions are better lovers, better husbands, and better fathers. Many women understand this and make an effort to teach the man they are close to about themselves in order to prevent antagonism between the sexes that is caused by wanting to be understood while doing nothing to further that understanding. And these women find that men really respond to their frankness and really want to learn about women. The fact that works in favor of this is that the people of Western culture have a deeply ingrained *tradition* of reverence and respect for women, and it is logical that this tradition should evolve new forms based on the better understanding of life gained by science.

Because of the new scientific understanding of childbirth, it is becoming more possible for a woman to bring the husband into the birth process. It is true that birth can be both painful, bloody, and sometimes frightening, but science has made it safer than it has ever been before, making it possible for women to want to share the joy that also comes with birth with their husbands. Today many women want to bring their husbands into the childbirth experience because they *need* them there and know that, underneath it all, there is an equally deep need in their husbands to be there. Which brings us to myth number three that denies that there is a paternal instinct.

The Myth of the Missing Paternal Instinct

From my own personal experience and observations of other men, I can attest to the fact that there is a male instinct to have children and to share the experience of childbirth with a beloved woman. Having had younger brothers and sisters, I grew up caring for infants and children. My mother was a registered nurse who made every effort to instruct me in childbirth, the facts of conception and embryology. But even though I had these advantages, like most other men of my generation, I was not allowed to help with the labor or witness the delivery of my children, despite the fact that I wanted to. And because of this, I felt that I was being denied something that was my right as a man and a father. I truly felt a sense of loss of a very important life experience. Later, when I was finally able to witness and assist with labor and birth, I *knew* for sure that the feelings that I had had before were both true and natural and, what is more, necessary to my mature development. I say with full assurance that childbirth is not only the greatest human experience, but one of the finest experiences that a man and woman can share. The instinct that makes a man yearn for direct involvement with the birth of his children brings him close to the creative principles of the universe.

Birth is one of the great mysteries of life, and no one can really ever fully comprehend it because it is both infinitely complex and divinely simple. I don't think that anyone can claim to be a fully mature human being in our time, without having witnessed birth and pondered upon all that it involves. Birth is something that we all want to know about from our earliest beginnings of consciousness. All children ask the question "Where did I come from?" The odd thing is that you can never really understand even the most graphic explanation of the facts until you have had the actual experience. And the reason for this is that there are emotions involved in the actual contact with birth that can never be explained in words or on film.

The need to *experience* the answer to this question is of very great importance to an adult male because it involves the satisfaction of an instinctive yearning. Man's desire to know his wife on the deepest level is fulfilled by sharing the experience of childbirth with her. The infant is *their* creation and *their* link with creation in nature, with the human past and the human future. I have observed these things in the interaction of couples in childbirth. And from having shared these experiences with them, I can say that something *within me* was also fulfilled, which I had felt had been forever lost to me.

Actually, I could have arranged to observe childbirth many years before I finally did, just as I was able to arrange to study medical anatomy for the needs of my professions of sculpture and morphology. But I could never bring myself to make the request to witness childbirth. The reason for this holding back on my part had to do with the fourth and biggest myth of childbirth—that of violent birth. Not until Leboyer broke this myth was I willing to observe the birth of a baby.

The Myth of the Necessity for Violent Birth

The most powerful myth surrounding childbirth—the one that has, above all others, separated husbands and wives from each other during the time of labor and delivery—is the myth of the necessity for violent birth. This myth is deeply ingrained in our past.[The myth that it is woman's lot to bear her children in loneliness and agony and that she is responsible for originating sin is one of the most tragic absurdities ever palmed off on innocent men and women and their newborns. The most dreadful part of it is that it has perpetuated the idea that women must suffer in childbirth and infants must come into the world with a scream of agony and a curse upon their innocence] This has prevented us for thousands of years from learning that labor and birth can be the most gentle, divine, and sacred experience possible. This myth of violent birth has been mankind's curse for five thousand years.

Because of this myth, women and infants have had to suffer painful and violent birth until fairly recent times. And this structuralized, rationalized violence has driven many kindly and caring men away from the process of childbirth with a sense of helplessness and grief.

The first break in the armor of this myth came in fairly recent times with the invention of obstetrical instruments, the discovery of the causes of infection, and the development of anesthesia. These developments of medical science made it possible for frightened and contracted women to have safe, medically supervised childbirth. These developments of medical science, which have taken place in the last two hundred years, gave the first great challenge to the old myths of violent birth and provided a secure period from which science could make the new observations and discoveries about the real nature of childbirth fear and contraction that have led us to the new era of scientific natural childbirth.

It is very important to stress here that natural childbirth is based on the discoveries of science and that it is only possible because medical science has developed to the present state of efficiency. I say this because there is a tendency for people to think that natural childbirth is a return to old, unscientific ways. Actually, there are five major discoveries in obstetrics and psychiatry that have enabled science to develop the new approach to natural childbirth—discoveries that have enabled us to finally see the old myth of violent birth for the curse it actually was.

Grantly Dick-Read was the great singlehanded pioneer of natural childbirth. One of a few neglected and unsung geniuses of this century, a man of infinite courage, fortitude, and human decency, he fought the battle for natural childbirth alone . . . against the trends of the entire medical profession . . . and he won the battle! He was a man's man, a superb athlete, keen lover of nature, and vigorous outdoorsman. But he was just as much a woman's man: He loved, admired, and respected women, worked his whole lifetime to understand them and find ways to aid them in the process of childbirth. He discovered almost all of the functions of what is now known as the natural childbirth process. There is not one positive development in natural childbirth that has occurred since his time that his research or practice did not touch upon.

His discoveries emerged from his inner faith and contact with nature's laws; he innately understood that childbirth did not have to be an experience of pain and sorrow. He saw early in his life that painful childbirth seldom occurred in nature outside of humans. These insights and his faith in the great design led him to find out why childbirth had become an unnaturally painful process.

He discovered the "fear-tension-pain" syndrome of childbirth. This discovery evolved through his observation that fear in childbirth leads to muscular tension which, in turn, leads to contractions so severe that they cause undue pain; this pain then increases the fear and promotes further tension, and so on. He went on to discover the physiological and neurological basis for this process. He then developed a technique that dissolved childbirth fears through prenatal education, prenatal exercise that promotes yielding, and breathing and relaxation techniques used in labor. His first book *Natural Childbirth*, based on over twenty years of research, was published in 1933.

The first major psychiatric insight into the problem of childbirth was made by Otto Rank, an early associate of Freud. Rank published a book called *The Trauma of Birth*, in 1923, which began to focus scientific thought on the emotional effects of traumatic birth and their relationship to the development of neuroses.

Many important discoveries that amplify and confirm Dick-Read's theories were made by another great, lonely, and tragic scientific pioneer, the psychiatrist Wilhelm Reich (who was also an associate of Freud). Among other things, Reich discovered the phenomenon of muscular armoring. This discovery was made as a result of his study of the process of character formation and the biological roots of neurotic character traits. Reich discovered that neurotic character traits result from emotional traumas that become fixed within the organism as patterns of chronic muscular tension. He found that these neurotic character traits can be dissolved when the bound-up emotional energy held within the armored musculature is released. He developed a therapeutic technique for releasing this bound-up energy in the musculature. These discoveries of Reich's were of major use to Leboyer in the development of his technique for dissolving the tensions in newborn infants with the use of the warm bath.

The fourth advance which followed on the coattails of the pioneering work of Grantly Dick-Read was made by Fernand Lamaze, a French obstetrician. Lamaze practiced orthodox obstetrics until 1951, when he went to the U.S.S.R. and spent five months at the Maternity Clinic of Nicolayev, in Leningrad. On his return to France he opened a clinic, using an approach to labor control based on Pavlovian techniques. His concepts took root largely because of the breakthrough made by the singlehanded efforts of Grantly Dick-Read, Lamaze being an adapter rather than an innovator or discoverer. His approach does not have the emotional, philosophic, or scientific depth of Grantly Dick-Read's, but it can be easily learned. And the great thing about it is that it brings the father into the childbirth processes, allowing him to work with his wife with the breathing patterns and help her stay in conscious contact. Lamaze is one of these strange scientific anomalies, an adapter of ideas who becomes more famous than the great pioneer-discoverer.

These developments finally brought us to the point where it became possible to discard the old myths that separated husbands and wives in childbirth and prevented them from sharing the greatest experience of life.

But there was one more important discovery yet to be made. This had to do with the way the infant is brought into the world; it has to do with the vast realm of emotion and sensitivity that in the newborn infant is so open, so tenderly perceptive, and so totally vulnerable.

Frederick Leboyer's book *Birth Without Violence* describes the technique of childbirth that Dr. Leboyer developed, with the most keen insight into the feelings and needs of the infant undergoing the process of birth. The fifth great discovery of childbirth has created a revolution in human understanding of what the newborn infant really is. In simple, deeply emotional, and poetic words, Leboyer has opened up the vast world of infant feeling and has, in the same simple terms, described the most loving and natural way to bring an infant into the world without shock or trauma (this will be described in detail further on).

All of these discoveries have made the present movement of scientific natural childbirth possible and have given it a firm foundation. This movement has several phases of meaning for budding new families. Of first importance is the fact that there can now be a fully conscious experience of the birth by both infant and mother, which allows them to establish immediate emotional contact. Of equal importance is that there now exists a childbirth technique that considers the infant as a human being and can prevent the emotional shock and trauma of birth from setting up the armoring process in the musculature of the infant. And the third is that the new scientific natural childbirth enables the father to participate in the labor and delivery process and to give both his wife and newborn child his warmth, strength, and support.

The meaning of all of this for all men, in these times, is that we now have a better way to build the foundations of our families than we have ever had before. We now have the means for creating the closest and deepest family relationship with those we love and live to protect. For five thousand years, men have been excluded from the most important experience of life, and now we are able to both observe this miracle and to take active part in the process! The fact that this has begun, however, does not mean that the last great myth of violent childbirth is yet gone; this last myth will die a hard death, but it does mean that men can now begin doing their part in breaking down the barriers that have for so long separated men and women from the deepest family union of all.

The Greatest Human Experience

The greatest tragedy of our times is the failure and dissolution of the family. Every day we read in the newspapers, hear on radio, and view on television the effects of lovelessness in the family structure of our culture. If what we read in the paper, hear on radio, or see on television were the *whole* truth, we could believe that our society was coming apart at the seams. Fortunately, we now know that new and stronger families can be created. So in light of the new method of childbirth and family creation we have just discussed, we realize that what all the bad news means is that the old myth of violent birth is having its dying convulsions. The tragic news serves to continually remind us how very important this new way of building families is for our time. It also makes it easier to understand that making sure that childbirth and the creation of a family are done in this better way is the way that each man can take responsibility for the future. Birth is the most important human event! It may not make headlines, but each birth that occurs is more significant than any other event that might be taken up by the news media. Each birth is a continuation of the whole creative process of the galaxy; it is part of a chain of events so vast that it boggles the mind to even attempt to follow it.

Men can take an active role in the process of childbirth, and it is well worth our while to reflect on the vastness of its meaning because we now have some new responsibilities, new things to learn, and new tasks to perform. There is a whole set of new realtionships that have come out of the development of the new scientific natural childbirth process: There is a new relationship with your wife, a new relationship with your newborn child, and a new kind of relationship with doctor, midwife, nurses, and hospital.

A New Relationship with Your Wife

One of the most remarkable things you will learn in observing the Leboyer method of natural childbirth is that there is an amazing transition from the pain of labor to the joy of birth. Seeing his wife undergo this transition teaches a man a tremendous respect for the courage and fortitude of women . . . their ability to endure pain for the promise of joy and fulfillment. So one of the major things you must understand will be happening is that your wife will be teaching you some lessons about her kind of grit and courage during labor and birth. You will learn, through participating in the birth process, a greater and deeper respect for what a woman is and, while this occurs, you will become more defined as a male and more naturally manly. But this new understanding does not come about by observation alone; it also comes about through your interacting with your wife with whatever techniques you use to help her ease the pains of contraction.

The new relationship really begins, long before the delivery date, when you learn the methods of alleviating the fear and pain of labor contractions. You learn how to breathe with your wife and she with you so that you work as a sensitive team together. In this breathing work, you can get to the stage where you almost feel that you are one organism. You will also learn what the three periods of labor are, how the contractions vary in each of them, and how you change the breathing patterns to handle the different kinds of contractions. And you will learn that you must bear the strong emotions of childbirth right long with her, feel what she feels, and be really in tune with her, in order to be able to guide her away from fear and pain.

This means that you will be learning to keep a very close emotional touch with your wife through eye contact—a soft looking into one another's eyes. It is necessary for you to learn how to do this because there is a tendency for people in fear or pain to blank out their visual contact which lets the pain take over. So by keeping this close visual contact with your wife, you help her to keep in touch with her courage. She can also draw strength and courage from her contact with you and know that she is not alone and that you are very special and important to her. You, better than anyone else, can help her in this way if you learn how to go about it.

The feeling of pain itself is caused by sharp and severe muscle contractions triggered by fear, and because of this, there is still another way that you can help your wife through labor. You can learn how to ease the contractions in some areas of her body by massage. Some people are naturally good at massage and have an instinctive ability to know just where to rub and just how much pressure to apply to relieve aches and pains. My mother was very good at it and my father had large strong hands that radiated very strong energy, so perhaps this is why I have a natural talent for massage. But I have also found that most people have a hidden talent for it and can be taught to do it very well with patience and practice. Practicing massage together is an excellent way for a couple to relieve everyday tensions in one another and is a wonderful comfort and aid for the woman during childbirth.

The basic principle of massage is to give warmth and movement to a muscle or muscular group so that the contraction is released. There is always a feeling of the muscle *letting go* when the tension dissolves, and this lets you know that you have done the right thing and lets your partner tell you that you have done the right thing. The easiest way to learn it is by practicing on each other and telling the other person where the tension is and how to go about rubbing that spot: "Work softly, rub harder, up, down, to the right . . ." is just about all you have to say. And if that doesn't work well enough, you can demonstrate on her what it is you want, or she can show you. The main point is to establish a kind of communication of touch.

The Grantly Dick-Read and Lamaze methods stress working on the lower back and abdomen as the major tension points, but you can also add your own variations with the massaging of shoulders and neck, spine, thighs, calves, and even the feet. Also, you can add further to your skills if you learn a bit about muscular anatomy (my own abilities were vastly increased by my study of anatomy). Whatever you are able to do in massage will help your wife immensely because she will then be able to tell you how to help her through her pain. It will also show her how much you *feel for her*, and that she is not alone.

A New Relationship to Your Newborn Infant

Along with the opportunity to form a new kind of relationship with your wife comes an equally new kind of relationship with your child that starts right from birth. At this point, you might not know very much about infants or have had much experience with them, and you may feel that you don't have much of an organic basis for understanding them. You probably think that because your baby has grown inside your wife, it is really she that the baby will care the most about. This is true to some extent, but not altogether, because there is an aspect of the development of the infant in the womb that has never really been considered and is very much in your favor.

Science has learned that in the womb the unborn child is full of feeling and that the embryo perceives all of the emotions of the mother as well as sensing the presence and emotions of people in her immediate environment. Because of this, there is no doubt that if you have been close and affectionate with your wife as the child has developed within her, the baby has experienced your presence as a very special human being. And what is more, all of the deep outgoing feelings that your wife has felt for you as she has carried the baby will be associated by the baby with the sense of your presence. I have seen a newborn infant respond to its father's embrace and touch in such a way that I cannot doubt that this special bond of love exists for the father who has been lovingly close to the mother during the embryonic development. So you see, you may have a great deal more going for you than you ever imagined.

What is there for you to know about babies? Is there some special knowledge required of you? No, nothing very special is needed at all except for you to realize that they have a tremendous ability to feel and sense your emotions. During the days of the old myths, people used to say that newborns didn't have important feelings, but now science has learned that they are immeasurably sensitive to the people around them, even before birth. This is why Dr. Leboyer's method of delivering babies makes so much sense and makes so very much difference in the emotional stability of the baby long after birth. This gentle approach to childbirth allows and encourages the contact and exchange of feelings between the mother and the baby and the father and the baby. You will be able to hold your baby in your arms and show it your love right away. And you may experience that very special infant smile of love and recognition. What do you have to know about babies? Only that you hold them in a gentle, confident way and that they *like* being held very much, just as grown-ups do when they are being loving.

What is really important is that you want to hold that baby and protect it with your body warmth. The baby will feel the warmth of your hands as your sheltering, protective fatherly love. You don't have to jiggle it or make strange sounds—the warmth of your hands is what counts, as well as the warmth of your chest. It's that simple.

The thing to remember is to be gentle and soft and not make abrupt or startling sounds and movements. A lot of people jiggle babies and bounce them up and down out of anxiety, but you should try to let the baby experience its own rhythms. Before you do anything to the baby, ask yourself whether it is something you'd like to be done to you if you were little and relatively helpless. Give your baby a chance to feel and respond to your breathing and body rhythms (you can do strenuous sports together in a few years). Let your baby feel calmness.

Another important thought about your relationship to your baby has to do with the general tendency of us men to be constantly proving ourselves and *acting* manly. There is more than one way for a man to show his strength and protectiveness, but the only way that a little infant understands is through your showing tenderness and gentleness. They *know* that you are big and powerful compared to their tiny defenselessness, so when you are soft and gentle with them, they feel that the power of your large organism is shielding them from harm, but when you are harsh or hard, they feel that it is directed against them. For an infant, comfort means being soft and relaxed. The only thing we men have to prove to our newborn children is our ability to be soft and gentle with them.

A New Relationship with Doctor, Midwife, Nurse, and Hospital

One of the problems you will face when your wife goes into labor will be your relationship to the doctor or midwife, nurses, and hospital. The reason for this is that you don't have the same kind of closeness to them as you have developed with your wife. Their functions and feelings about the birth of your child are somewhat different from yours. They are practitioners of medical science, and science involves formal procedures and strict adherence to rules. This means that hospitals are a little like law courts, police stations, or the army, because they have to be run according to the book or they just won't work efficiently. So the only way that you are going to make certain that you and your wife will have the best experience possible is for you to become familiar with the hospital layout of labor room, delivery room, and recovery area, as well as the hospital childbirth procedure. The idea is for you to learn where you will be, how you will be able to move about, and how you can concentrate your thoughts so that you and your wife are most at ease. Your childbirth class should teach you all this, and you can obtain additional information from your doctor.

Next, you are going to have to work under the guidance of your doctor or midwife and the hospital nurses. They are there to ensure that everything goes safely and smoothly for your wife and newborn, but they will not be too concerned about you. This means that you can only expect a good relationship with them if you have learned your childbirth lessons well and have established very good communication with your wife. If you have learned enough about labor and childbirth and are able to work as a team with your wife, the doctor and nurses will recognize this and let you take on as much of the responsibility as you can handle. Your rights as a father will only be measured by the amount of responsibility you can take on. If you can help all the way through labor, with emotional contact and breathing teamwork with your wife, help her communicate her needs to everyone, and at the same time co-operate in the hospital procedure, you will be doing your full job. But if you are not able to manage some of these things, you will have to stand out of the way, on the sidelines, while someone else takes over the things you can't do.

What you have to understand is that doctors, midwives, nurses, and hospital can take over the whole process of childbirth and leave you to stand aside as a passive observer because they are trained to manage childbirth efficiently and safely. But the things that they cannot do are the things that your wife and you can do together with deep emotional contact. So you see, the creation of this new kind of family actually depends very much upon you in the end. If you learn how to handle the childbirth situation, no doctor, midwife, nurse, or hospital can give your wife and newborn child the special kind of support and love that you can. No one but you will have the necessary motivations, emotional needs, and basis for contact with them.

Though birth is the most important event of life, without your participation, medical technology can make it a sort of production-line process. Doctors and nurses do have feelings of reverence for birth, but they have to get on to the next job, and because of this, it can never be the big event for them that it is for you. But they will help you and your wife to have the most meaningful experience of your lives if you show them that you have done your homework.

HOW THIS BOOK WAS BORN

The reason for my doing this book has to do with your right and duty as a father to know the motives and values of *anyone* who may affect the life and development of your child. Your becoming a father means that you will be responsible for the protection of the life and development of your child, so you have every right to ask who I am and why I think that I have something to tell you about childbirth.

The writing of this book emerged from my study of the Cycle of Life. As a sculptor, I have been working on a long-term project of creating a Cycle of Life chapel, containing sculptures that depict human beings in the most important ages, moods, and relationships of life. To prepare for this work, I have had to learn everything I could about the forms, relationships, and feelings of life. I have been making studies of the human family for over twenty years. It has been necessary for me to study anatomy, embryology, psychology, movement, character development, and history. In the course of this study I have also earned a doctorate in the field of morphology—the study of form development.

The hardest task of all has always been to learn what life is really about beneath surface appearances. This has required a serious amount of self-criticism and questioning about how much I really know about all the things I have studied. Eventually this process of self-criticism led me to face the fact that I was ignorant about one of the most basic aspects of life—birth. Even though I was a father who had been interested in embryology and child-birth for years and had been around many newborns and become known as a sculptor of the human family, I had to admit that there was something missing in my understanding of birth. There was something basic missing from my knowledge of the newborn. But what seemed more peculiar to me was that it was not facts that were missing; what was missing was more a matter of how the facts were understood. I felt something was wrong in the basic approach to the newborn and that this "something wrong" in my own understanding was also wrong in the whole society.

Feeling the depth of my own ignorance depressed me because childbirth is at the very center of the Cycle of Life. I felt that I could not honestly continue my Cycle of Life project unless I somehow learned what birth was really about. This realization brought about a serious emotional crisis in which my entire life's work seemed threatened and my whole future looked very doubtful. I felt that the extent of my ignorance was so basic that all of my previous work with the Cycle of Life might not be valid and this added to my depression.

You can imagine how I felt: There I was, in middle age, feeling that my whole life had gone down the drain, that I had spent my adult years with the illusion that I was a sculptor of the Cycle of Life when in reality I didn't know the most important aspect of my subject. This was hard to take, but I had a core feeling of blind faith that I had been on the right track, and this core of faith grew a little stronger when I realized that the ignorance and the depression that seemed to come from it was anything but unique. It dawned on me that many men in middle age experience a crisis and depression. I began to wonder what it was that we all shared in common. More of the pattern became clear.

Middle age is a time when a man either moves on to a higher stage of maturity and functioning or finds that he has spent his life following false values and empty dreams. During this time of life, many men in our society become severely depressed, and some even die, unless they can emerge from the self-evaluation feeling that life is full of new and hopeful things. These *new and hopeful things* seemed to me to be the key to it all. It is important to have the feeling of having done worthwhile things, but it is *even more* important to have the feeling that life is good at the very core, and at the very beginning.

It was helpful for me to realize that the depression I was experiencing was a common experience, a thing that might possibly be necessary for my own further development. "Why shouldn't I question my own worth and values?" I thought. "*Has* my work had the depth and feeling that the Cycle of Life project should have?" Serious self-questioning seemed positive and right, and I realized that being able to ask these questions was reason enough to keep on working and trying to solve the problem of the missing factor in my understanding about birth.

Going through this period of questioning was as difficult as anything I had previously experienced in my life. I ruthlessly examined every value and concept. During this time, I also studied more intensely and tried to get closer to the understanding of the whole process of birth in nature—the for-

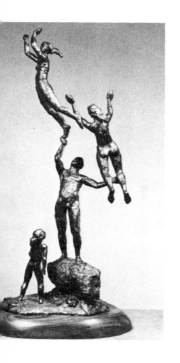
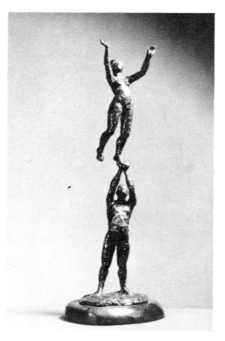
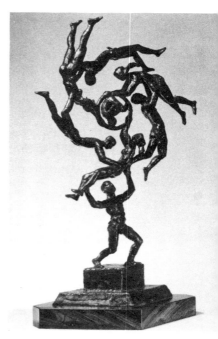

mation of galaxies, cell division, embryology; I looked into nature as deeply as I could. This was good for my spirits, even though I frequently felt that I was getting no closer to the answer. Actually, this intensive study prepared me and enabled me to see the key to my problem when it finally appeared. I'm sure that I would have overlooked this very simple thing if I had not worked at opening myself up to the whole problem of birth in nature. What finally helped me turn the corner was a picture of an infant in a magazine—a newborn infant with a heavenly smile on its face. Millions of people saw the picture, which had come from a simply and beautifully written book *Birth Without Violence*, by Dr. Frederick Leboyer.

This picture was an illumination to my mind and emotions; it removed a tremendous weight from me. I clipped it from the magazine and tacked it up on the bulletin board in my studio; it delighted me. It wasn't that it told me anything exactly new about the newborn infant, but rather that it told me something I had always dimly known. It was full proof that life at its

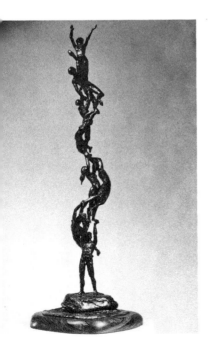
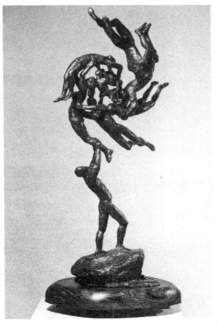
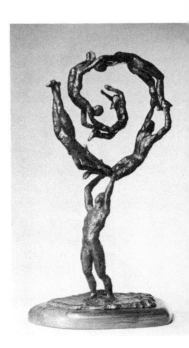

beginning can be joyous, full of boundless, radiant feeling. This newborn infant's expression was easy, effortless, flowing, spontaneous, and full of natural good nature. It made me realize that the trouble caused by the human race is created by not letting life be, by interfering with life through some kind of dread that causes violent striving and straining in people, fighting to *try to get* feeling instead of allowing feeling to come by itself, losing faith in life. But there it was, all joy and loving hope, in the face of a newborn baby. I wondered whether the millions of people who saw the picture had experienced any of the feelings I was having. This picture changed my life.

Why was I so moved by this photograph? Why did it have the power to change my life? For many years, from the time I began to think my own thoughts, I had felt that all the capacities for feeling and thought are right there in each new human infant at birth. I understood that we don't *learn to feel* or *learn to think* so much as we merely expand the huge potentiality

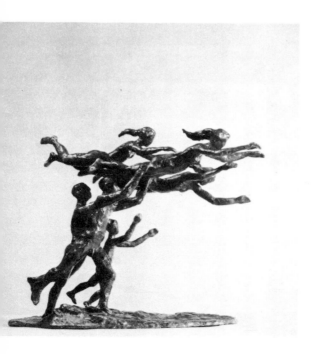
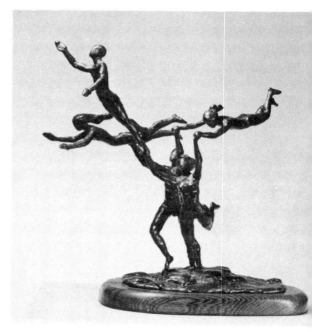

that is within us at birth. Instead of having no feeling or thought, the new-born infant holds within itself all feeling and all understanding in potential so that teaching should be a matter of guiding development rather than forcing concepts into infants and children as though into empty containers. I had known this in a vague and instinctive way; the feeling that it was true had always been the roots of my faith, had somehow sustained me most of my adult life. But when I saw the smiling infant, I *consciously knew* that what I had felt all these years was true and that my instincts about the Cycle of Life had always been correct: My life's work had not been wrong after all! What had been wrong was the culturally implanted image which tells us that coming into this life is of necessity a matter of suffering and agony, a basic primordial cry.

Mankind can be basically good, decent, loving, and hopeful *at birth!* Once a person can see this, the understanding quickly follows that the things that go wrong with life, the dreadful things that human beings do, are the

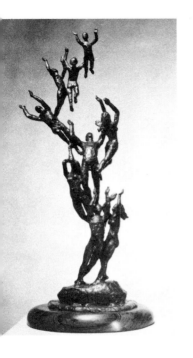 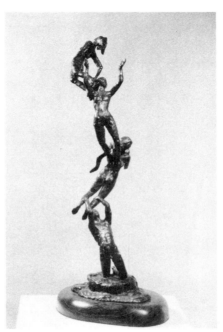 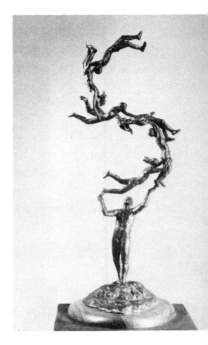

result of shock and damage to their emotions as infants and children—traumas that knock the joy and hope out of them. This realization made *me* see that it was terribly important for humankind to have new images of life that show what life at its best can be. Not only did my Cycle of Life project appear valid in its basic affirmation of life, it seemed vitally necessary! It was a way to protect what I saw in that newborn infant face, a way of showing people what is there within infants, waiting to be born.

I had a powerful personal feeling about that infant, a feeling that made me want to protect all infants from ever having their capacity for joy and loving radiance destroyed. This feeling made me want to help guarantee that human infants be given a chance to come into the world without having their spirits broken by the brutal administration of harsh slaps and mechanical treatment that is passed off with the excuse that "they can't really feel anything."

That was my reason to go on living and working; I had found the central meaning and motivation of my Cycle of Life chapel. I felt that I had also gained an insight into these depressions that are so common to middle-aged people in our society: The burdens of life seem much heavier and less worthwhile when people feel that life begins and ends in grief. When people believe this, they feel that the basic expression of life is suffering and tragedy. This becomes all the more painful when the person senses that he or she has been robbed of the capacity for joy.

I think that underneath it all the life force within a person always knows that the joy could have been there. Because of this, these depressions that come in the mature years are the result of life's central image having been twisted and distorted—the reason for the distortion being an unsolvable riddle or cruel joke of fate. Who could know otherwise when the image of birth, as seen for thousands of years, has been of a frightened shrieking infant born of a half-agonized and frightened mother?

Lacking in human experience has been *the recorded visual image* that proves that joy and love are possible and natural at birth. Even though I had sensed that this joy could be a basic part of family creation and had expressed this in my work, my own feelings that this was true had been gradually worn down by the cultural imagery of trivia, hate, violence, depersonalization, bitterness, and contempt that is projected in the movies, on TV, and in publications. Even in the field of fine art, which is supposed to be the reflection of society's highest hopes and values, the human figure has been ruthlessly distorted, emotionally twisted, and emptied of all human feeling. I am not sure whether one's feelings of the affirmation for life *can* withstand the continuous assault of these negative images. Even I had come close to feeling that my dream of a Cycle of Life chapel was the foolishness of an aging man, a man who probably did not have the kind of ruthlessness necessary to survive in a basically cruel existence. And the truth is, I wouldn't have really wanted to survive if I had come to feel that life at its core was cruel. The infant face changed all that for me.

The infant face showed me the truth about human nature and it made me want to dig my heels in and fight for that truth against the imagery of ruthlessness, violence, and distorted feeling. It showed me *what to fight* as well as *what to fight for*. It made me feel that it is worth fighting against any odds to help the newborn, even when strength is gone and the task seems impossible. It showed me that *manhood-gentleness-fatherhood-strength*, though separate words, have to be blended all together to make a man worthy to live in the great spiraling Cycle of Life. It had taken the image of an infant child to teach me this!

Why is it that we have never before seen this smiling infant face? For five thousand years we have accepted an image that told us we are basically sinful by nature, possessing drives and passions that must be crushed in us when we are still infants and children. The insane part of all this is that it has been the crushing of infants and children that has produced distorted drives and passions in the adults! Distorted images of life have perpetuated the sinful treatment of mothers in childbirth and their newborns. These sinful images have told us that mothers must experience fear and pain in labor and that infants must scream with their first breath. These sinful images have separated husbands from the right to comfort and ease the fear of their wives in labor and from embracing their newborn infants at the *time when they most need one another and can be most truly united!* These are the things that this little infant face told so clearly. It also said that we humans can be splendid at the very beginning and that we must all work to make this so.

I don't want to give you the impression that I was sitting in the corner waiting for the end to come during the time I was experiencing this crisis. Though I felt despair, I kept on working, and though there was a feeling of instant relief and illumination when I first saw the picture of the infant, the changes followed slowly. One of the first things that came about was a wordless determination to see that kind of infant joy at firsthand. After reading *Birth Without Violence*, I decided to try to arrange to travel to France, to see Dr. Leboyer and gain permission to observe childbirth with his patients. But this did not come about. As they sometimes do, things worked out in a quite different and surprising way.

How I Met Dr. John Grover

When people look for ways to survive times that are difficult emotionally and spiritually, they frequently search their memories of childhood for images of happier days. One of the things that helped me through my emotional crisis was fishing, one of the joys of life that my father had shared with me. My father was fun to fish with because he had a way of leaving me alone to learn for myself, but he also had the knack of coming by and putting a little pressure on at the exact time when it was needed.

Being with him was always a great pleasure to me, no matter what we were doing. He was a happy-go-lucky man who could create fun out of nothing. When I was a child, my father was the greatest man in the world. He gave me warmth that has stayed with me all my life. After we had been standing at his bedside during the time he was dying, my sister Marjie told me that she had never seen so much love in anyone's face as she had seen in my own for our father. I have no way of knowing what she saw, but I still think my old man was the best that ever lived. He was surely no saint, but he had a zest for life that stayed with him right to the end. Many months after I had begun writing this book, I remembered that my mother had told me that my father had been with her when I was born. I cannot help but feel that this had something to do with the very special love I had for him. And it is my hope that this memory of mine will show you how very important you can be to your own child.

It was natural for me to turn to fishing during my time of depression because it was a way of bringing back my father's supportive love. It worked too: I started fishing again to recapture something that I'd lost and ended up becoming a far better fisherman than I was when I was a kid. It was through fishing that I met Dr. John Grover. I had gone to Manchester, Vermont, in the fall of the year of the infant picture, to learn about fly-fishing. I attended a three-day seminar run by an outfit that makes very fine fishing rods and equipment. I felt that the challenge of learning a new and difficult way to fish would dispel the last of my depression before I finished up some work and traveled to France to see Dr. Leboyer. I found that I really liked fly-fishing; in addition, the classes were interesting and my fellow students bright and engaging people.

One of these people was a rancher from California whom I liked right away since I am a native Californian and had experienced some ranching life in my early years. He was a rugged, straightforward sort of person and I enjoyed our conversations during breaks between classes. One evening I

came into the dining room of the lodge a little early, before the lights had
been turned on, and in the dim light I sat at a table next to a man I thought
was this rancher. I said "hello" and went on to ask whether he had decided
to purchase a very fine bamboo fly rod that he'd been looking at that after-
noon.

"I think you've mistaken me for someone else," the man replied. At that
point I saw that I had, although this man had the same sort of brawny,
manly quality of the rancher. I explained the reason for my mistake to the
stranger and we fell into conversation. It turned out that he had just come
in from an eight-day hike up the Appalachian Trail. When we got around
to occupations, I told him that I was a sculptor, working in the Cycle of
Life tradition, and then went on to ask, "What do you do?"

"I'm an obstetrician," he replied.

"That's a field that I am very interested in," I said. And then, through a
sudden impulse, because the Leboyer technique is controversial in the obstetrics field, I asked, "Do you by any chance know anything about the
Leboyer method of delivering babies?"

"Yes," he answered. "I do it."

Things in Common

There are times in life when events seem to be guided by forces and
currents outside myself with a greater purpose than I can quite understand.
Whether I call these occurrences the result of chance, fate, destiny, or the
pattern of a great design, they are often events that open up whole new directions in my life. Sometimes I am aware that these things are taking place
and sometimes I am not, but the evening I met Dr. Grover I could not help
feeling that the great designer of life had sent this man to me, and I knew
beyond doubt that I had passed beyond my crisis and was on the way to

something new. I knew that this man, Dr. John Grover of Boston, Assistant Professor of Obstetrics at Harvard Medical School, practitioner of the Leboyer method of childbirth, would lead me to that smiling infant face that I had been searching for.

Trying to stifle my feelings of awe and revelation, I set about doing everything that I could do to convince Dr. Grover that I was a sincerely interested and worthwhile individual who could learn something of great importance from him. I told him more about my Cycle of Life sculpture project. He in turn responded with more facts about his own work. Then I went on to tell him of my desire to observe childbirth and the reasons why this was important to my work.

At that point in our conversation, I remembered that I was scheduled, the following month, to give a lecture on my concepts of morphology (the science of form) to a group of artists and scientists at Harvard. I mentioned this, hoping that it would give us some opportunity to meet. I also told him that I would like to send him one of my books. During the course of our conversation, I was hoping that I wasn't putting him off by my show of enthusiasm and that he did not feel that the Cycle of Life sculpture concept was another example of the craziness that exists in the art field.

When the meal was over, we exchanged addresses and went our separate ways. Later that evening I wrote a note, giving him a little more information about my scheduled lecture.

When I returned home a few days later, I sent the book I had promised him, with a letter reaffirming my interest in his work and Dr. Leboyer's concepts. A week later, I received a reply from him that added more dimensions to my feelings about the forces of destiny. The letter told me that, in the early 1960s, Dr. Grover and his wife had visited Oslo, Norway, where he was very taken with Gustav Vigeland's great sculpture park. (Vigeland was the Norwegian sculptor of genius who singlehandedly founded the Cycle of Life tradition in art.) A few years later, his wife had bought him a book that had come out on Vigeland's life and work. This happened to be *The Embrace of Life*, my book on Vigeland's sculpture. After he had returned home, Dr. Grover realized that I had written this book.

This coincidence was important to us both because it enabled us to see that our interests in human life were closely linked. After this, it was easy for us to work out a plan to meet in Boston. We agreed to do so to discuss how to arrange my observation of babies being born.

Losing and Winning

The Harvard lecture was a disaster. For many years, I have been a professional lecturer and know my fields of sculpture and morphology as well as anyone, but it was like running full tilt into a brick wall. This was a meeting of two diametrically opposed directions of thought, which was particularly difficult because I sensed no friendly presence in the entire audience. The only thing I was aware of was a wall of malice and coldness. As shocking as this was to me, in the light of my feelings about the Cycle of Life, my failure to achieve communication with this particular group of artists and scientists proved to be useful to me.

There were some distinguished scholars in morphology in the audience and their opposition meant one of two things: that they were right in their approach and I was wrong or that I had an approach to morphology that was completely new to them. Realizing how long it had taken me to understand Cycle of Life concepts, I saw that I could not convince anyone in such a brief time. This meant the lecture was doomed to be a failure. The odd part about this realization was that it gave me a sense of total confidence. I have never seen quite so clearly that if science and art are to serve life, rather than enslave it, they will have to be based on knowledge and feeling for the human Life Cycle. The evening was put into perspective for me when at the end of it one of·the scientists said that they were work-ing at creating *"machines that feel just like human beings."* He then asked me what I thought about that. I answered that they would do well to think about what the feelings of life *really* are.

You will see, during the course of this book, that the differences be-tween these contrasting ways of thinking have very much to do with the way we live our lives and the way children are brought into this world. The difference between my views and those of my Harvard audience pointed up the differences between the kind of science and art that aims at defining *and* furthering human functions, feelings, and concerns, and the kind of mechanistic science and art that aims at abstraction as its *ultimate goal.*

My trip to Boston was a marvelous practical demonstration of the differences between these two directions: On the one hand there was the Harvard audience, with whom my feelings and views were in conflict, and on the other there was Dr. John Grover, who was about as warmhearted and humanly concerned with the things I care about as a man can be and to whom I seemed to get closer the longer we talked. But as John is also a member of the faculty of Harvard (Medical School), I assume that this proves that neither viewpoint has yet won the battle. All in all, I felt I had won far more than I had lost.

What Kind of Man Is Dr. Grover?

As you read this book I think you will have realized that the basic un-derlying premise is that human feeling is the most important aspect of the whole childbirth process. What I mean by this is that your life, your wife's, and your baby's can only be linked, outside of the heredity factor, by your mutual capacity to feel emotions within yourselves and in the other family members. This interdependent emotional circle is what makes you a family and the thing that enables the experience of family life to move all of you through the various stages of the Cycle of Life.

So it follows that an important part of the task of the people who are involved in helping you with the birth of your baby is to help you all to establish and protect these links of feeling among the three of you. Seeing that your baby is born safely, and that your wife goes through the birth process safely, is only a part of what should happen during the birth. Many doctors are beginning to adopt this broader view of the birth process, and to my mind, Dr. Grover is one of the finest examples of this new kind of *family-centered* obstetrical physician. Because I feel that it is important for you to understand the kind of person he is, I'd like to tell you some of the things I have come to know about him.

To begin with he's a man like you and me, having a certain number of good points and a certain number of failings. The main feeling that I have of him is of a steady, extremely dependable, extremely good-natured person.

When I first met John, I had no idea at all that his standing in his profession is very high; that I had met a doctor who used the Leboyer delivery technique and that there were so many natural links between us, after having been brought together in such an unusual way, was quite startling enough. I guess I was quite surprised when I later learned just how eminent a man he is, since he doesn't act the role of the eminent doctor but is just a straightforward, kindly person.

I have learned from having studied the development of natural childbirth that the men who have done the most for women and infants, and have advanced the art of childbirth the most, have been pretty rugged and masculine types. Grantly Dick-Read, the founder of the natural childbirth movement, had been a championship boxer, horseman, a crack shot, and an ardent fly fisherman-naturalist. Wilhelm Reich, the discoverer of muscular armoring, was probably the most vital man I have ever met. There seems to be something that is very natural and virile in the deep concern with child-birth.

I spent a lot of time with John Grover and saw him under fire in situa-tions of stress that were almost impossibly trying. And it is at just these times that the real man comes to the fore. At these times I've experienced an awed feeling for his utter dependability. And each time that I have been with him for any length of time, I have experienced a strong feeling that I am with an extremely *fine* human being.

John Grover cares about life and he particularly cares about newborn life and young mothers and fathers. I think that if I can say that I am a Cycle of Life sculptor, I can also say that Dr. Grover is a Cycle of Life physician. He is a man who has a feeling for the whole spectrum of life, a man who has "reverence for life."

During our meeting in Boston, we worked out a general plan for my study of childbirth. I was to come to Boston three months from that time, to observe babies being born and devote at least a month to the task.

How to Observe a Baby Being Born

After I had returned home, it began to dawn on me that there was a basic research problem that I had not even considered. It's one thing to *talk* about observing childbirth, but it's something else to figure out *how* to do it without standing there giving the impression that you are gawking at other peoples' private affairs. At first sight this might not seem like much of a problem, but young couples are not too keen on having strangers intruding on their most important feelings and experiences, and hospital officials don't like people wandering around their precincts, rubbernecking and getting in the way. I realized that it would be difficult for people to accept that what I really wanted was to watch babies born out of their mothers' bodies for the sheer curiosity of it. Yet the truth of the matter was that this was exactly what I wanted to do! I wanted to find out what the feelings involved in this experience would be. I had no idea of *what* I would discover or feel. All that I really knew was that this was something that was very important for me to see. I knew that seeing it would be incredibly important to my life and work, and it has proved to be true beyond anything that I had imagined.

Dr. Grover understood that I could not quite explain why I was doing this study. I was perfectly honest with him about not wanting to come to the project with preconceived notions. I had no particular intention of doing a sculpture of a child being born or of writing a paper on the morphology of pregnancy. I felt that the mother, father, and infant would teach me *something*, but I didn't know what. I sensed that this something might effect a change in me that would alter my whole outlook rather than produce one isolated piece of sculpture or one academic article. So with Dr. Grover's guidance I wrote a research proposal that was acceptable to his professor and the authorities of the Boston Hospital for Women. Thinking back, I realize that their acceptance was extremely generous since my proposal was very open and not what is usually regarded as scientific.

Nevertheless, to make doubly sure that I would not be thrown off the delivery floor if someone objected to my standing there simply looking, I decided that the best way for me to create an aura of acceptability would be to take along my camera. There is something about a person holding an expensive camera that gives others reassurance, even though he might actually be just standing there looking. It turned out that this, originally unintended, use of camera became a very important part of the project and led directly to the writing of this book.

When these technical matters were settled, it remained for me to figure out the kind of relationship I would be having with Dr. Grover's patients and their husbands. The big question I asked myself was, "What right have I to present myself to young couples having their first babies, asking whether they mind very much if I stand and watch while their baby is being born." It seemed to me that such a request coming from a stranger would be unpardonably rude, and I just didn't want to commit that kind of intrusion on anyone. I wondered whether there was any legitimate way for me to present myself to the young couples and obtain, not just their permission, but their enthusiastic consent for me to be with them.

Pondering this problem, I realized that the only way it would work for either me or them would be if these couples liked me and had some sympathy with my need to know about childbirth. And I realized, also, that this might come about if I told them about myself, my work with the Cycle of Life project. One thing was certain: I did not want to have a cold and impersonal experience with these couples. I felt that if these couples accepted me, they would be sharing something unusually special with me and this sharing had to be done with warmth and friendship. The only flaw in this condition was that there was no way of knowing if warmth and friendship would occur with any of these particular people.

Why Personalness Is Important

Right about now I can hear you asking yourself, "Why is he dwelling on all these personal matters, his crisis of middle age, his father, his feelings for Dr. Grover, and the feelings he wants to have with the couples? Why doesn't he just get on with the problems of childbirth?" The answer is quite simple: Childbirth is the *most* personal experience of any of the experiences of life. This feeling of *personalness* is the most overwhelming *feeling* about childbirth. But it isn't separate personalness, it is open and shared personalness where each person is distinct, yet all are drawn together. It has been found that we all relive our own births over and over again throughout our lives. Birth is the first great formative consciousness experience, where you cease to be a part of your mother and enter the world of voluntary separateness and voluntary sharing.

You will find that there is nothing abstract about birth when your child comes. The birth of your baby will reach right down to your core and to the core of all those who participate. Birth, more than anything else, makes us realize that we do not live life by abstractions. To living creatures, nature's laws are personal: Energy, gravity, air, water, sunlight, and growth are all very personal facts of survival and feeling to every living creature.

On the level of conscious life, the things that mean the most to us are the personal things—the human contacts and experiences that come to us in our passage along the Cycle of Life. We love most those who are related to us by birth or close association—wives, husbands, children, parents, friends, and workmates. Birth calls up all of these personal feelings because birth itself is a great act of sharing.

Once I realized the importance of this personal factor in birth, I was able to go to Boston to meet Dr. Grover's young couples. I had found what would make it work. And this is why it *did* work.

This feeling of personalness will be important to your wife, your baby, and you in your own experience with birth. When the time comes, you will want the people who will be with you to care very much about your wife's feelings, your baby's, and your own. If you do find people who can care for the three of you, *their* feelings will, in turn, add to the whole experience.

To Boston

On the evening of my arrival in Boston John and Philipa Grover were ready for me, with a gathering of parents-to-be. A second gathering was held at Dr. Grover's offices on the following day for couples who lived farther away.

In all, there were ten couples who were expecting their first babies within the coming month. On both occasions, Dr. Grover showed two films that had been made of his delivery techniques: the first made before he began to use the Leboyer method and the second one after he had learned it. Following the showing of the films, he gave a talk to the expectant parents about what would be happening during the labor process and how mother, father, and doctor would be working together during the birth. When this was over, he introduced me and I made a few remarks about my interest in childbirth and the Cycle of Life.

On both occasions I found the couples to be very attractive and bright people. All of them had attended childbirth preparation classes and had learned the Lamaze technique. The Grantly Dick-Read approach was not mentioned.

At the first gathering, the reactions of the couples to the possibility of my observing the birth of their babies were quite startling to me. The responses ranged through hostility, skepticism, and indifference to guarded interest and enthusiasm. I was totally unprepared for such a wide spectrum of feeling. At the end of the evening, I was in a mental turmoil trying to figure out the reasons for such a wide variety of responses.

As I lay awake thinking about what had happened that night, I realized that even though I had wanted to be accepted by *all* of them, I was asking something of them that they had no obligation whatsoever to grant me. These people were, quite rightly, concerned with having the best possible conditions for the birth of their babies, conditions they could cope with. So if that meant not having me around, I was in total sympathy with them. I felt that what I had interpreted as hostility was probably only very strong anxiety about privacy and the fear that my presence would cause unwanted complexity. I even felt that the couple who expressed guarded interest would probably do better if I was not there. Nevertheless, I was a bit depressed because one couple out of six was not a very strong statistical average. That thought might almost have made me overlook my one success if the people involved had been a little different.

The enthusiastic couple, Susan and Larry, had utterly charmed me. They were delighted at my interest in childbirth, thought it was terrific that I would be with them taking photographs, and were fascinated by the fact that I was an artist. They gave off such sparkle, such warmth, confidence, and acceptance that I was overwhelmed. I was as puzzled by their acceptance as I was disappointed by the rejections of the others. You'll be hearing a lot more about this couple, and I think that you will learn, as I was to learn, what wonderful and extraordinary people they are.

Before I dropped off to sleep that night, I thought about each of the couples I had met. I had really liked *all* of them very much. They had all been honest with me in telling me their feelings. Each couple had taught me something valuable, and I felt that they had helped me to grow more emotionally that night than I had in years. But as I drifted off, thoughts about Susan and Larry kept recurring to me . . . their responsiveness . . . their vitality. Maybe they could teach this old sculptor a little something more about life!

The Second Meeting

By the time the meeting with the next group of couples took place the following morning, I had put my thoughts together and felt that I could meet the new couples with a lot more confidence than I had felt the night before. Particularly useful to me was the realization that what I had interpreted as hostility the night before was an expression by the men of a very fundamental kind of concern for their wives and as yet unborn infants, for their privacy and family integrity. Realizing this enabled me to approach this new group with much greater tact and understanding. I made up my mind to try to compensate for this natural fear by stressing that privacy was something I felt very strongly about. I also realized that there is an element of the husband's feeling left out in the whole aura of childbirth, and I decided to stress my feeling about the man's role a little more strongly.

As we drove to his office, Dr. Grover was very silently supportive. He seemed to appreciate that I was really working to understand the problems I was experiencing. He didn't say very much, didn't try to tell me what to do, but seemed to be letting things take their course in a natural way. Realizing this, my confidence in him grew by leaps and bounds.

At this second meeting, I did a great deal better in expressing my purposes and feelings, and I also told them about my own disappointments at the birth of my own children. As a result of this, three of the four couples present said they wanted me to be with them when their babies were born. And the declining couple was able to reject the idea without any feeling of pressure or resentment. My spirits rose considerably.

The three couples were each strongly individual and interesting. They expressed their feelings about my being with them in strikingly different ways. Eric spoke in a very firm and warm way for his wife, Laura, and said that they would like to have me with them. Bob and Debbie were quiet and gentle in their agreement. My new friend Lillian, on the other hand, spontaneously walked across the room, and we spontaneously hugged each other while her husband, Oscar, looked on with a twinkle in his eye and a certain measure of good-natured skepticism. Later on, Lillian told me that Oscar had said, "Who is this guy? Are you sure you want him with us?" as they were leaving the office. "Sure," she said. "There's something I like about him, something *simpático*."

Getting to Know the Parents-to-Be

My next step was to get to know these young couples better and learn something about their lives and feelings. Dr. Grover and I had planned that I would come to his office daily, to get a feeling of how he related to expectant mothers and to give me a chance to see my own special mothers, whenever they came to his office for their checkups. But as this seemed a limited way of seeing them and I was left with a lot of free time, it occurred to me that I could ask each couple if I could visit them in their homes so that we could get better acquainted. In their own surroundings, they were sure to be more relaxed and comfortable. It was also just as necessary for them to get to know me as it was for me to know them. I wanted them to feel relaxed with me too; my instincts told me that this was a *very important* goal to achieve.

However, the most immediate problem for me was to find a place to live that was near enough to Dr. Grover's office for me to get there quickly. After searching the papers and getting nowhere, I finally found a room in a roominghouse through a referral service that Massachusetts General Hospital provides for visiting researchers.

Soon after I was settled and had familiarized myself with the route to the office, I began making visits to my couples. It didn't take me long to realize that this was the best possible way to get to know them and was the smartest move I made during the whole project. *They* were in *their* element and putting *me* at ease. It was truly remarkable to see the pleasure they took in the fact that I was honestly interested in their experience of childbirth. Their generosity of spirit and sharing was so beautiful, it made me think that the doctors who have stopped making house calls have unwittingly cut themselves off from real contact with their patients and from half of the pleasure that is possible in the doctor-patient relationship. During my stay, I was able to visit three of the couples in their homes but missed one couple for a very good reason.

I did not visit Debbie and Bob because their baby was due last, and I felt that I had plenty of time before the birth to arrange the visit. Naturally, their baby was the first to arrive. They were truly disappointed that I had not visited them in their home, and Debbie expressed this disappointment to me quite a number of times. Of course, I did visit them later, but it was not quite the same as it would have been before. It was this that made me realize just how very important these prebirth visits were: A kind of sharing is involved that can be had in no other way. Fortunately, I had seen Debbie several times in Dr. Grover's office. I talked with her the day before she went to the hospital and did feel that we had reached a very warm friendliness.

The conversations that I had with the couples in their homes were free and easy. We talked about the things we liked to do and about ourselves. I was interested in knowing where they came from, what kind of work they did, how they had become acquainted, and all sorts of details of everyday life. They seemed to thoroughly enjoy telling me about their lives. As I listened, it often occurred to me that there was something important that linked us all together—them, myself, and Dr. Grover—it was the feeling of human confidence. We seemed to be building links of trust between us, links that would help us through whatever uncertainties each of us felt. In this building of confidence, Dr. Grover seemed to be the central figure, and this made me realize how important the role of the doctor can be in terms of the emotional as well as the technical aspects of the birth process.

There is a certain amount of natural anxiety involved in childbirth and being an emotionally responsive person, I spent a lot of time anxiously waiting during that month. I seemed to be always slightly on edge, knowing that any minute of the day or night the doctor's buzzer machine, which I carried attached to my belt, might go off. One time it did go off in unusual circumstances.

I was sitting in a theater watching a very good movie that was just drawing to the climax. It buzzed. I shot out of my seat like an arrow and rushed to a phone to call the central office for instructions as I'd been advised to do. I fumbled for coins, nervously dialed, waited for the voice that would tell me who was delivering and when I should dash to the hospital. It turned out to be John who "just wanted to know if the buzzer was working." I confess to being completely miffed for a moment or two, but then the humor of the situation struck me and I had to laugh. I suddenly saw good-natured John Grover at the other end of the telephone, and I began to visualize all the movies that had been interrupted for *him* over the years, all of the parties, vacations, and the nights of sleep when he'd just begun to doze off and that blasted buzzer went off for the real thing as well as numberless false alarms.

Just to add a bit more to the anxiety factor, there was the thought that the buzzer *might fail to go off* for some reason. And, lest you think that this was the anxiety of some sort of a Nervous Nellie, there finally came a time when it didn't work when they were trying to reach me.

I became totally submerged in the phenomenon of birth. Every day at John's office I would get it from some new angle because either Dr. Grover or his partner, Sheila Lynch, would hand me another book on childbirth, inquiring whether I had read it or not.

The expression "giving birth" seems to apply to the emotions of all people who surround a birth. The coming of an infant brings out the feeling of giving in everyone when things are right. I know that I felt the urge to reinforce the confidence of my young couples in whatever way I could. We had some good conversations about fatherhood, and I think that we all agreed that it was important for men to learn to show their tenderness and warmth to their newborn infants, to be closer to them and to their wives.

I suppose I felt myself to be fairly well prepared for what was to come. I had been a father myself, been around newborn babies, had a keen interest in embryology and birth, and had once worked as a surgical attendant in a big hospital during my student days. But despite all this, I was not prepared for the full impact of the emotions of birth. Birth is a great and powerful human event, with a depth of meaning that we can hardly fathom. I was soon to experience some of the most profoundly moving events of my entire life.

ERIC AND LAURA

Even though I missed being with them at the birth of their baby, I learned things from Eric and Laura that are most important to our discussion of fathers and childbirth. The fact that I actually missed this particular birth was the factor that, in the great design of things, enabled me to understand what they had to teach me. Their baby came later than was originally expected, beyond the time that I had set aside for my stay in Boston. I *could* have stayed longer, but something within me told me that I had already learned something very important from Eric and Laura. The trouble was that I didn't know what it was, and it took me about a year to understand their lesson.

When I visited them in their home, they served me a dinner fit for a king, and to my surprise, much of the meal had been cooked by Eric. This led me to the discovery that, in addition to pursuing his graduate studies, after his service in Vietnam, Eric had gone to work in a fancy restaurant. Starting as a waiter, he went on to become chef and finally ended up managing the place (while continuing his studies). This gives you some idea of the kind of capability this man possesses. Not only was the meal superb, but it was made even more delightful by Laura's wit and charm.

Laura is a person who bubbles with a sense of playfulness and delight, the kind of woman that children adore. She teaches music to children and is herself an accomplished singer. I found her to be lovable and friendly.

They were the first couple I visited. Being a bit apprehensive about whether Laura would really accept me, the thing that impressed me right from the beginning was the way she made me feel, from the moment I walked in their door—that I was not just a friend but a fully accredited member of the childbirth team. When we first met in Dr. Grover's office, I hadn't noticed her reaction to me because I was so beguiled by her general quality of openness. But meeting her in her own home left no doubt that she had made a place for me at the birth. She gave me the feeling that she really *wanted* me to be there. It was my reflection on this wonderful openness of hers that awakened my realization that women in childbirth *need* the attendance of people who care about them as individuals. This feeling of welcoming that she gave me was even more strongly understood when I had missed the birth of their baby and had returned to Boston to visit them at the hospital with Dr. Grover. That day both Eric and Laura told me in positive terms that they had actually missed me.

Oddly enough, *I* did not feel too disappointed about missing the birth of their baby! This wasn't out of disinterest in them either, because I had an enormous amount of feeling for them. Dr. Grover, Eric, and Laura all told me how things went with the birth and that they had talked about me, and I realized that, in a sense, I *had* been there. It was slightly confusing, but thinking about it over a long period of time enabled me actually to realize what it was that I had learned. The lesson had to do with the kind of man that Eric is. It finally dawned on me that I had felt that Eric is the kind of man who is totally equipped to participate in the birth of his own child.

It was a big step for me to understand why I had such great faith in Eric. He is important to this study of childbirth because his personal qualities as a man are those that are necessary to any man who wishes to take an active role in the birth of his children. We can think of these traits as being the newly evolving qualities of fatherhood.

Eric is a fine-looking, erect man who sports a great handle-bar mustache, a hold-over from his service as a front-line medic in Vietnam. I think the mustache may have been originally grown to cover his sensitivity and youthfulness at a time when he had to take on some terrifically tough and dangerous responsibilities. The face and the man have long since matured, and strength and experience are there to carry off any kind of facial decoration he might choose. However, there is nothing of the swaggerer about Eric; he doesn't act any part; he's a straightforward, honest man.

Eric is no braggart; he made no attempt to dramatize himself. But in the simple way he told me of his wartime experiences I realized that he had been through several years of violent and bloody action and in the course of his service had, as a matter of routine, helped many young men like himself survive. An interesting sidelight of his Vietnam experience was that he also delivered several Vietnamese babies in emergency situations.

If I've learned nothing else from my years of studying the Cycle of Life, I've learned to recognize a good and decent man when I see one. This is a man who gave his loyalty and service to saving lives while under fire, and he doesn't make a big thing of having done it. He simply did what was needed at the time and has now moved on to do the best job he can at whatever he meets in life. He isn't a professional veteran, and he could care less about following the medical profession in civilian life; he's a man who meets life's challenges. I believe that this is a quality worthy of the deepest respect, and what is more, I believe that it can be found in many men. This is the quality that makes fatherhood.

I don't mean to imply in anyway that men have to be tested for manliness under gun-fire. I simply mean that courage, loyalty, and devotion are the qualities that we must bring to our wives and newborns in childbirth. And as fathers, we should nurture these qualities within ourselves.

I realized that these qualities that Eric possesses so generously were the source of my respect for him. He is the kind of man you would want on your side if there was trouble, or the kind of man you would like as a neighbor. When he talks, his words make sense; when he works, he gives the best of himself. He is a man whose word you can trust as well as being a man who likes a good hearty laugh. Sensing all this about him was why something he said, as we were having dinner, stayed with me for a long time afterward. He said, "Nathan, there isn't any book that really *talks* to men about childbirth. I looked for one, but I couldn't find one."

I am not altogether sure that Eric ever really needed a book to tell him how to be loyal, strong, and supportive. He has these qualities in abundance and so do many of our fellow countrymen. But it was that chance remark of Eric's that first planted the idea of this book in my mind, even though I did not realize it till sometime later.

BOB AND DEBBIE

The forces of nature are vast and powerful beyond our comprehension, and the conception, embryonic growth, and birth of a baby are as much a "cosmic event" as any of the acts of creation that take place in our galaxy, but we humans often fail to recognize that birth is a part of this whole continuum. The recognition of the forces of creation in the birth of Bob and Debbie's baby was quite overwhelming. The birth of this baby taught me that even though we might feel we are prepared for birth, the experience is so powerful, so deep, and so wondrous that it leaves us feeling we can never grasp its whole meaning.

As I told you earlier, I was unable to visit Debbie and Bob in their home before the birth because their baby came three weeks sooner than was expected. As a consequence, I never got to know them as well as I might have, had I spent a convivial evening with them. Everything the birth of their baby had to teach me caught me off balance and knocked holes in all my preconceptions.

You will remember that I met Debbie in Dr. Grover's office the day before she rushed off to the hospital in labor and that this enabled me to begin to get acquainted with her. At that time, she told me something about Bob and herself, their life, and hopes for the future. During the time we were talking together, I was quite taken by a look in her eyes that I can only describe as being extremely gentle and *yielding*. This look of yielding was quite out of the ordinary and I couldn't understand its meaning. However, when I learned that she had been rushed to the hospital in labor the following day, I could not help but feel that the expression I had seen had something to do with her readiness to yield her baby to the birth process. So I was not too surprised to hear she had been taken to the hospital. Nevertheless, what took place afterward did surprise me, and the biggest surprises seemed to come from my own reactions to the birth process.

This was exactly what I first saw after rushing to the hospital with Dr. Grover; getting dressed in a surgeon's scrub suit, like the one Bob is wearing; and walking into the labor room right off the main area of the maternity floor. The central control area of the maternity floor bears some resemblance to an aircraft control tower at a busy airport: Nurses, doctors, and operating-room assistants move with brisk efficiency, patients' names and numbers are chalked on a big blackboard, and there is the general air of people trying to avoid mid-air collisions. I remembered that I used to enjoy this atmosphere when I was an operating-room attendant years ago, when I was an art student. But it seemed to me, this time, that it was not quite the atmosphere to enhance the kind of contact and mood that is sought in Leboyer childbirth—one of calm, quiet feeling and contact.

At least Debbie didn't seem to be all that comfortable about it when I first saw her. This picture seems to prove that nurses are more secure, comfortable, happy, at ease, and confident about being in a hospital than the women they attend in labor. On considering the reasons for Debbie's feelings of discomfort, I realized that she was being examined by a woman she had never met before, had been dressed in an unflattering garment that was not her own, was in a strange environment beyond her control that was totally unlike her home environment, also knowing that her body and feelings will be exposed to the looks and touches of strangers. A major fact I learned about Debbie later was that she does not like hospitals.

Debbie's face shows a certain resigned tolerance of the situation, while Bob's whole stance seems to say that he recognizes a lot of the things that Debbie is feeling and knows that he can't do much about them. But regardless of that, he stood steadfastly by his wife to give her every bit of comfort he could under the circumstances.

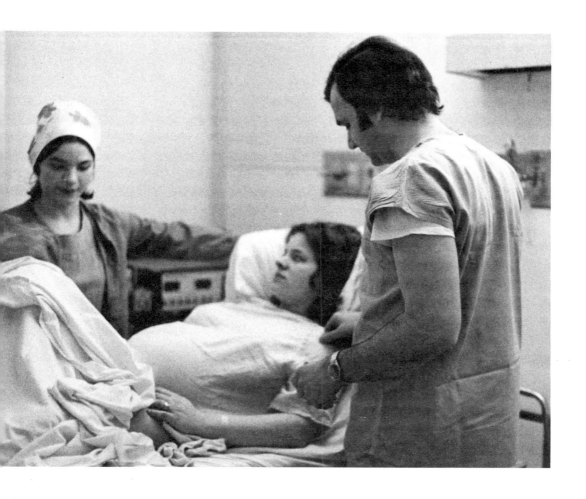

This was the emotional scene, according to my perceptions, when I entered the room with Dr. Grover, and my immediate feelings were those of an absolutely helpless intruder. At that time I didn't know Debbie or Bob well enough to have my presence mean anything to them in the way of support, but Dr. Grover's presence seemed to bring sunshine into the room and confidence to Debbie. Her spirits rose 100 per cent.

My first view of labor fear-tension-pain was anything but detached—it seemed to cut right through me; there is an emotional charge behind the expression of this kind of pain that is like no other. I believe that the basis for this is the fact that the labor fear-tension-pain syndrome emerges from anxiety for the genital-reproduction system and because of this comes from the very core of the woman. It can touch a man right to his depths when he sees it occurring in a woman and probably has the same frightful association to him as injury to the testicles. We men must mimetically respond to this agony when we see it with an echo of these contractions within our own bodies. Probably our first instinct is to take flight.

Dr. Grover moved right in there, giving Debbie assurance while he massaged her lower abdomen. I may have wanted to respond to her fear-tension-pain in some way, but felt there was nothing I could do. I almost fled from the room, feeling that the only decent thing I could do would be to *not intrude.*

I noticed that there was something rather self-righteous in this *noble* attitude of mine even then, but it took me several months to realize that, right at that time, I was "acting out" the historical role of the "helpless man" who has left women to suffer in childbirth for thousands of years. When I realized this later, I began to wonder what it was that blocked me from walking over to Debbie, touching her, and attempting to comfort her. What was it that prevented me from comforting a fellow human who was obviously suffering fear and pain? Was it my own genital fear, was it that I didn't know her well enough, or was it that I felt Bob might not understand?

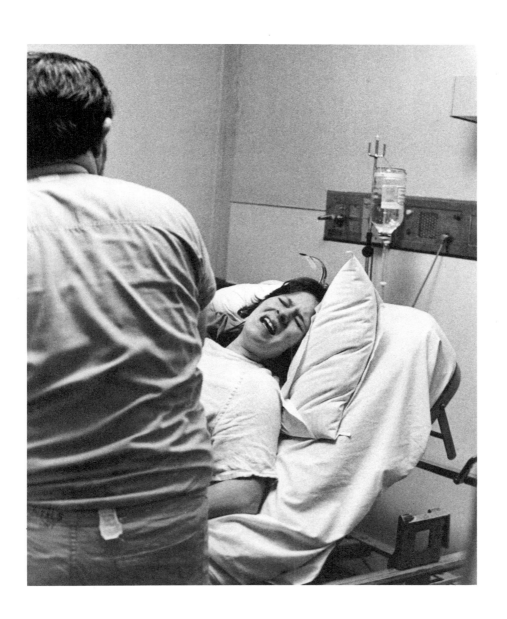

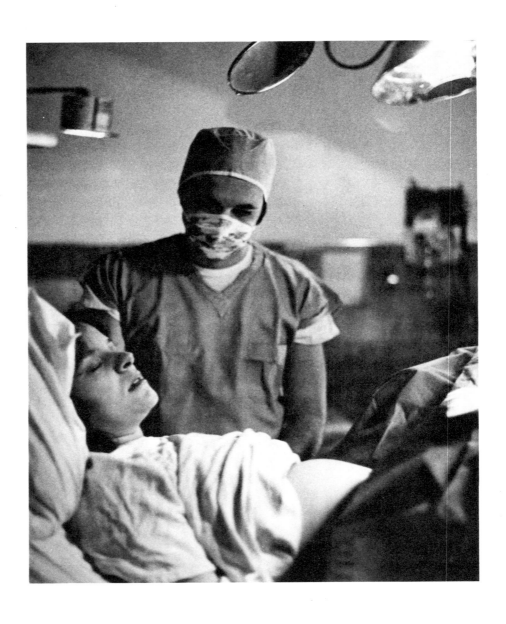

Whatever it was, it wasn't something that I alone was experiencing; *all of us* seemed to hold back except Dr. Grover.

I spent the next two hours in the doctors' lounge, experiencing a mixture of feelings because I was too "noble" to watch a woman in pain while, at the same time, I was full of natural curiosity about how the labor was getting on (with the inner wish that I could help). So I am not sure how well Bob and Debbie did with the application of the Lamaze technique, but from general impressions I received later, I gathered that everything happened so fast they were off balance and didn't really get into it. Debbie wasn't confident that she could handle the pain and so was given a saddle-block anesthesia: a local anesthesia which shuts off nerve impulses in the pelvic area and allows the woman to remain completely awake. Looking at this picture, you can see that Debbie carried a large degree of the burden of the labor within herself.

Both Bob and Debbie have a tremendous amount of feeling and capacity for contact, but the unexpectedness of things happening weeks ahead of schedule seemed to affect their teamwork, and there was Debbie's obvious discomfort with hospitals to put them off stride. But despite all that, *they were together emotionally* through their whole experience of labor, and whether the breathing techniques worked out well or not, you can see Bob's expression of concern for Debbie here, and she could see it, feel it, and sense it too.

Debbie's expression at this point made me feel that she had been driven to the end of her endurance, beyond being able to take any more. But as was soon proven to me, I was totally wrong and had no conception at all of her reserves of energy or the swift emotional changes that were about to take place in her.

The delivery room was darkened to protect the eyes of the newborn baby from the shock of glaring lights. The baby, having moved in the birth canal with its head "crowning," was just about ready to emerge within the

next few contractions as Debbie "pushed" her abdominal muscles down-
ward in an expelling movement.

What struck me here was how Dr. Grover dominated the whole delivery room at this point. Everyone was under his spell as the kindly strength
of his personality seemed to draw everyone's energy into the last efforts of
birth and not just Debbie's alone. It was much the same as in music when a
great orchestra conductor draws the finest efforts from his musicians in the
climax of a symphony. It was as though all Debbie's feelings of fear-tension-pain had given way completely from a self-centering toward a great
emotional expansion as the powerful forces of the birth process itself
gripped the whole room. It was as though we were all spectators at a miracle—even Bob and Debbie!

Here I noticed that strong and gentle feelings seemed to flow from Bob
to Debbie, and he seemed linked with his wife, giving her his support and
reassurance.

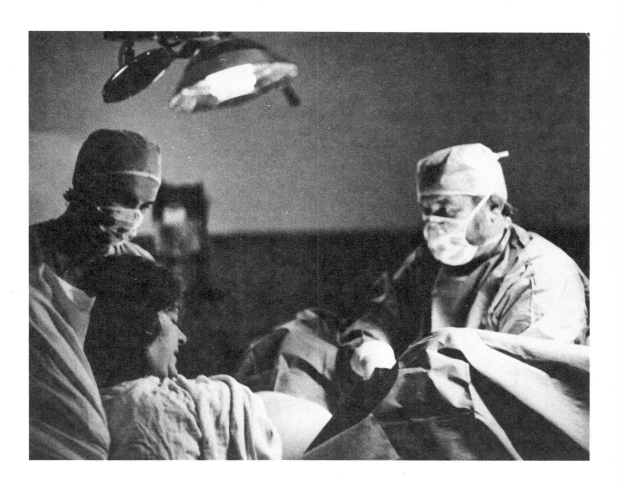

Birthing . . . the baby emerges so fast, so fast, a slippery, little human creature! One can hardly see it at first, but one can feel it because its presence fills the room and everyone's eyes and energy are centered on it. Everything is out of focus, everybody strains to see . . . the new life, the miracle . . . boy or girl miracle? There is a sense of people being astounded beyond any real capacity to ever totally grasp what has happened—the arrival of a new human being and the beginning of a whole new and unique human consciousness.

IT'S A GIRL!!!!

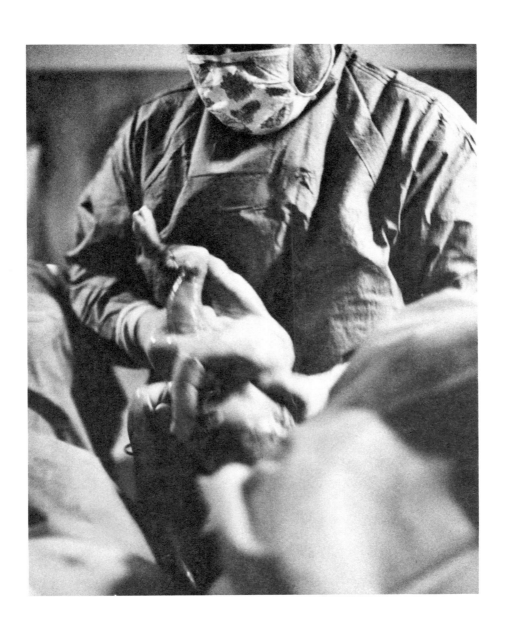

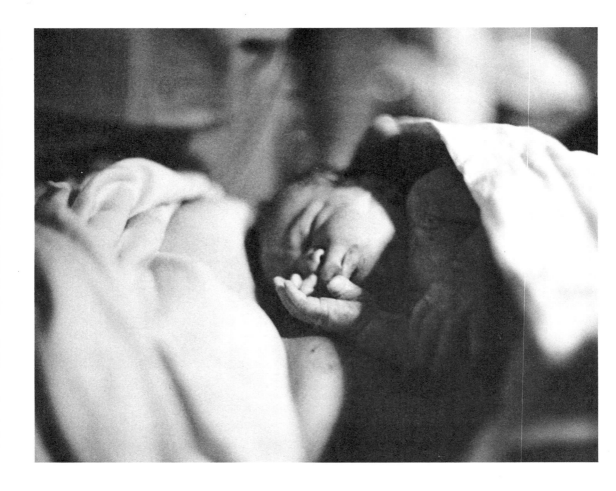

Everyone strains to see the baby which Dr. Grover has placed to rest on her mother's stomach. There is a feeling of people all around, but the odd thing is that their egos have completely submerged or disappeared for a moment, as though to allow the ego of the baby to emerge and expand. How closely everyone looks, how intensely eyes are focused on this little creature. But now there seemed to be an overwhelming tension growing and gripping everyone underneath everything else at this point, as though an incredibly important human question was being asked by the unconscious of everyone in the room.

IS THIS CHILD WELL FORMED?

I only realized the potency of this silent question much, much later. It was an organic question that emerged from our very energetic roots and genetic patterns: Is the infant strong, will it be able to survive, and most important of all, is it molded to the necessary human pattern? There is no getting around this underlying human concern for conformity. It is something that of necessity *has* to be lived through right after the birth itself. This is probably *the* single dominant object of underlying fear felt by all women giving birth for the first time. It is something that is just *there* as a possibility until the baby is born, until a woman can *see* her capacity to create a whole life. This was why there seemed to be a general feeling, which immediately followed this first successful passing of this test, that seemed to say: "Welcome home, safe and sound."

WELCOME TO THIS WORLD, LITTLE HUMAN PERSON!

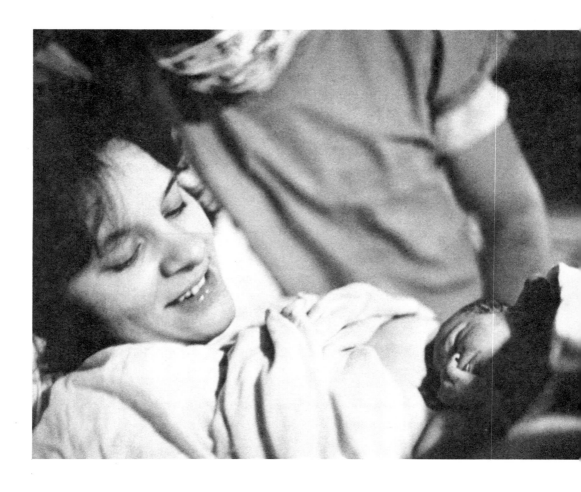

As Debbie held her baby on her stomach, I was conscious of her hand delicately, almost timidly, holding her child. She was experiencing this period of silence and withheld emotion. It was as though a brief flash of fear gripped her as it had momentarily gripped the other people in the room, the sharp awareness that something *could* be wrong with the baby, the sudden collected focus of the vague fears that must have come to her from time to time during her pregnancy that would have to be resolved at this very moment:

> FINGERS, TOES, FEATURES . . . ALL
> SO DELICATE,
> SO FINE,
> SO PERFECT . . .
> AND
> SO MIRACULOUS!

I have never seen such an astounding change in a woman's face and in a woman's emotions as I saw in Debbie's at that time, from seeming agony to actual joy. At that moment I began to understand a little something about women—the reasons for their capacity to shift so quickly in the range of emotional scale. As the gentle flood of love seemed to flow from this woman's body and face to enfold her baby girl, her husband was drawn toward them both with an instinctive urge to encircle them with his arms and body.

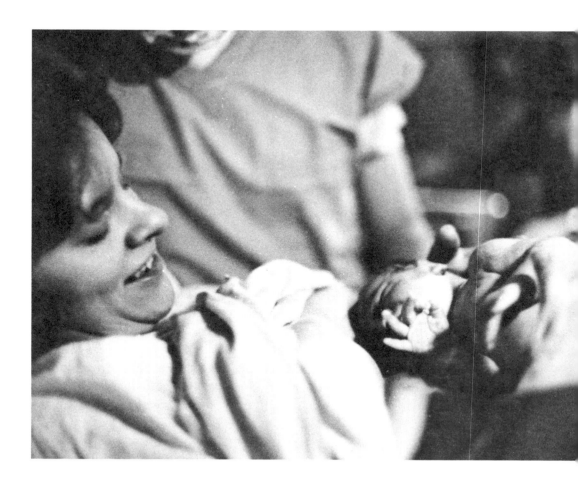

A SUNRISE RADIANCE BEGAN TO FILL THE ROOM

My immediate feeling at this point, I am ashamed to say, was a sting of jealousy and a sense of deprivation so deep that I almost couldn't bear it. For a brief moment I felt so totally forlorn and empty that it almost left me in shock. *I* had never had love like this. I had never experienced such tenderness and beauty. It hit me like acid, bitter and galling! What *I* had missed, how life had robbed *me!*

Then just as suddenly, as I continued to look at this rising, gentle radiance, I realized that the swift flash of bitterness was dropping away. Why? Because I was *part* of what was happening, because I was sharing it all. I realized that this beautiful thing that was happening to Debbie and Bob was happening to me too. The emptiness *had* been there, but now it was gone: I had witnessed the great miracle, and something indescribably forlorn had left me, dropped away forever.

All these feelings happened in an instant, and I seemed to let go of years of grief and puzzlement as the feeling with Bob, Debbie, and their baby swiftly grew in pulsing changes. Debbie's mood shifted from the first gentle flood of love and delight to a glow of confidence. And then, as though it was impossible to resist, Bob's hands reached to touch his newborn child.

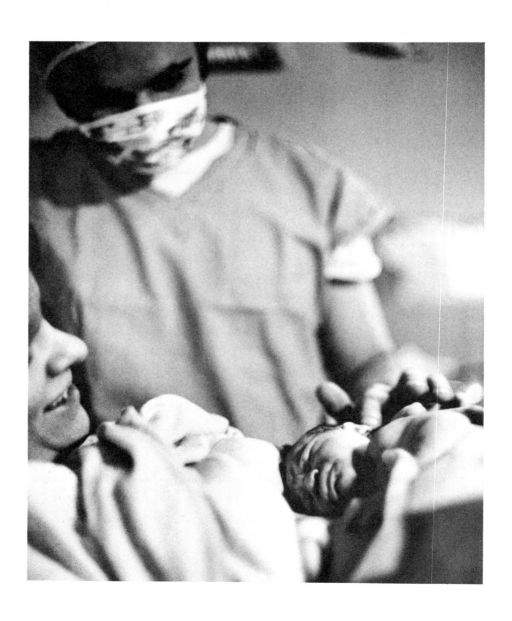

And with the first
gentle
touch of the new father,
that delicate marveling
deep from within him
for his woman's
infinite capacity to
share the arts of
miracle making,
one
two
three
became
one:
a FAMILY
had been born!

This shows an altogether private look from Debbie to Bob. She has an amazingly expressive face and this look seems to have more to do with the first phases of child creation than with the final birthing of the infant. But then again, it seems to say that the joy of lovemaking and the creation and birth of this infant are all part of the deepening of their feelings for one another.

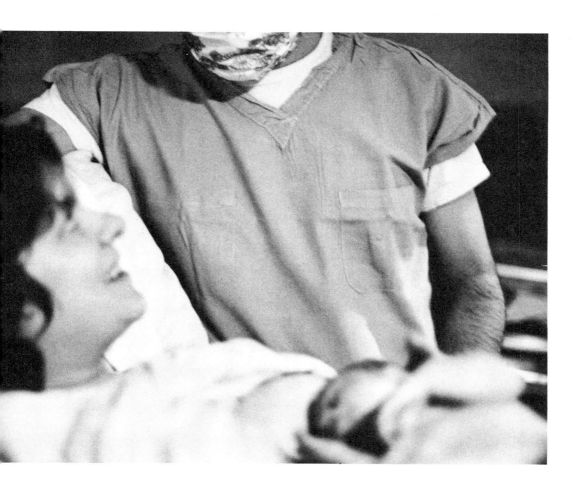

Whatever that unfathomable look that Bob and Debbie shared may have meant to them, and I suspect that it had a million nuances, it drew Bob and Debbie and their baby into a close circle. The people outside that circle remained respectfully silent and seemed not only to understand their being excluded from this intimacy, but to want to withdraw so that the intimacy could grow.

Through all of this, there was some movement in the background, but I felt that the presence of Dr. Grover was radiating a controlling influence over the nurses and attendants in the effort to give Debbie and Bob the silence and space for their feelings to expand and develop.

I could see that this was a very crucial time for the new mother and father, as it was their first experience of sharing the birth of their infant. I realized that just as it is important to bring the *baby* into the world with gentle and non-violent treatment, it is also important that the newborn *family* have the same gentle and non-violent atmosphere so that their memory images of the first few moments of the creation of their family will have the beauty and strength necessary to sustain them through whatever lies ahead.

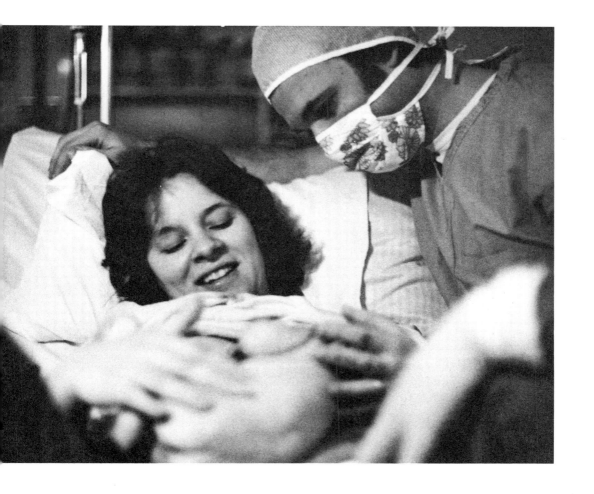

After the baby had rested on Debbie's stomach and the parents had had time to draw their emotions together, Dr. Grover was ready to cut the baby's umbilical cord, which by this time had stopped pulsating and pumping needed blood and oxygen to the baby. The baby was then put in the warm bath you see here, to rest again in the weightless floating state until it reached a state of total relaxation. This great innovation of Dr. Leboyer's long search to find ways to bring infants into the world with gentleness is an almost miraculous way for the baby to let go of any muscular tensions that may have come about through difficult aspects of its birth or traumatic events that may have occurred right afterward.

In the bath, the little newborn could be seen to actually let go tensions and begin to move its hands and feet rhythmically, and its little face lost its contraction of eyes, brow, and mouth; it began to open its eyes and awake from its desire to stay in its mother's womb for another three weeks.

During the time that Debbie had been separated from her baby, she had given birth to the placenta which Dr. Grover showed us all, calling it the "house" where the baby has been living. I found the placenta to be extremely beautiful in color as it had a range of colors similar to those in the glazes of Renoir's late paintings. He showed us the placenta because he wanted us to understand that it is a truly remarkable organ.

During this separation from her baby, Debbie had time to regain her composure and to build her energy. It was as if she realized within herself that she had done everything as well as she was able to and had come through with flying colors. It was at this point she said to me, "You know,

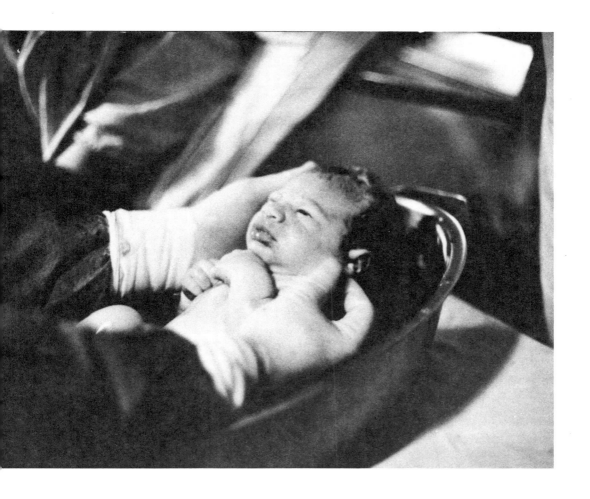

Nathan, next time I'll be able to do much better." I had the feeling then that what she was saying was that she would never again be so frightened by labor, that she knew now that she could take whatever pain was involved and never again be frightened by fear itself.

As all this was going on, Bob was having his own first experience of handling and caring for the baby as he helped Dr. Grover hold the baby in the warm water. Dr. Grover explained at this point that newborn babies are not yet able to maintain their own temperature, so the Leboyer bath also helps to regain temperature level.

After the bath had relaxed the baby, she was taken to special table designed for newborn babies where she was examined more thoroughly, her footprints taken, and a small band put around her wrist for further identification. Her umbilicus was treated and she was given clothing and medication was put in her eyes.

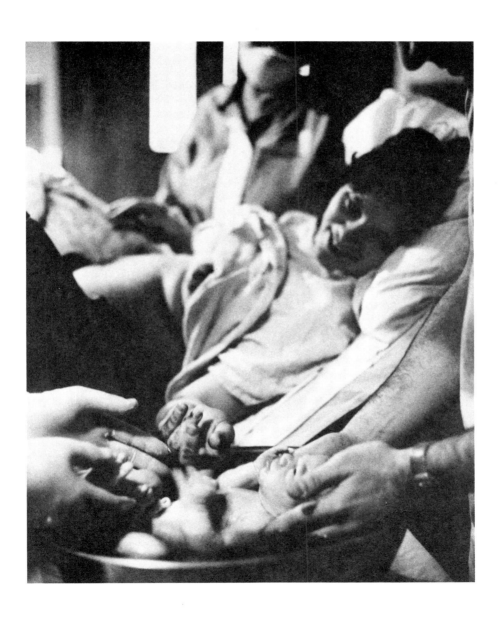

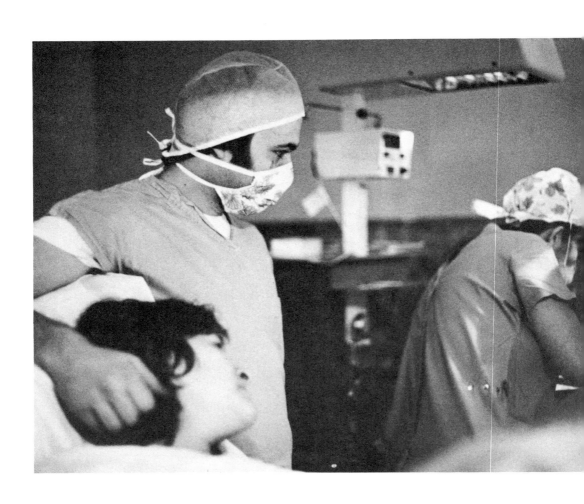

This abrupt separation of the baby from the parents seemed to be an intrusion upon their developing feelings, and what is more, it seemed a rather serious intrusion upon the developing feelings of the newborn infant. At this most crucial time, laws of both the state and hospital administrations are brought to bear on the newly born family by the rigid and mechanical enforcement of two laws that, though created for very sound reasons, can be rather shocking to the emotions of the newborn. These laws are rigidly enforced with no sensitivity at all for the feelings of the individuals involved. The parents are two sometimes frightened and always emotionally charged people, who are undergoing one of the most powerful and demanding of human experiences, and the newborn is a human being whose expanding sensory system has just emerged from the sheltering, warm environment of its mother's womb into the vast and frightening planetary environment.

The baby is, as they say in police circles, mugged, printed, and given an ID band by people who are not necessarily insensitive but do not have the powerful and flowing love and contact for the infant that its parents have. That, in itself, is probably somewhat terrifying to the newborn whose vast and open sensory system is capable of picking up absolutely every emotional nuance. This kind of mechanical contact can create a violent displacement of emotion through a misapplication of a very good rule, namely: Don't let the babies get mixed up in the hospital nursery. There is no question that identification is important but this ID work with the newborn infant *could* be done later when the emotional relationships with the parents have had proper time to grow.

On the other hand, the intrusion by the state with the mechanical application of silver nitrate ointment to *all* babies' eyes is highly questionable. In this situation the completely helpless infant, whose sensory system is both totally expanding and totally vulnerable, has a harsh and astringent medication forced into its *eyes*. Eyes are the organs that are most sensitive, most vulnerable, and most subtly important for emotional development during

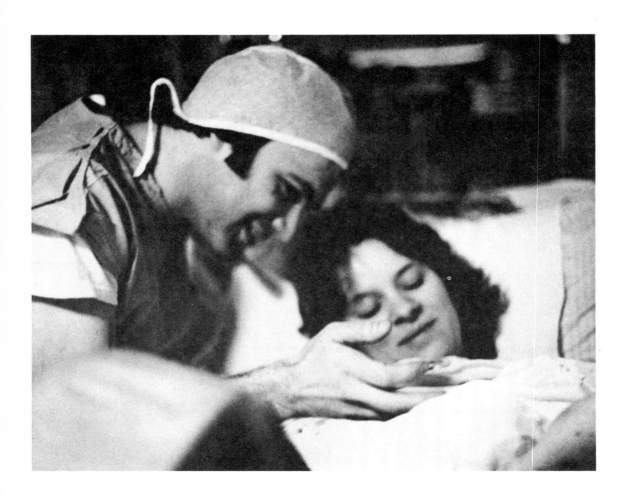

infancy (and for that matter during its whole lifetime). Our eyes are our only windows to the universe. So what happens? With this rigid application of a law (that is useful if applied correctly), there is created the greatest single violent assault on the newborn infant. It is tragic that this archaic practice from the old violent methods of childbirth is still retained and adhered to with such mindless rigidity.

The reason for the application of the silver nitrate ointment to the baby's eyes is for the prevention of blindness to the baby from infection by gonorrhea germs. A very sensible thing to do when applied to the newborns of people who *have* gonorrhea infections! But our objection to silver nitrate is absolutely valid when you learn that antibiotics can do the same job and are a lot less painful (if they are painful at all) to the baby's eyes. However, the sense of being in Kafkaland really increases, when you consider that silver nitrate medication is given to infants *whose parents do not have any infection at all!* The excuse for this is that it is too much trouble for the hospital to determine whether people do have gonorrhea prior to the birth. In other words, 90 per cent or more of newborns are given unnecessary violent pain and emotional trauma to their most sensitive organ of perception. This occurs because the people responsible for the safe birth and sound emotional development of newborns have not yet become sensitive enough to the sound of pain or agony in a newborn infant's cry to find ways to solve the relatively simple scientific problem of testing mothers for infection before birth.

The baby is returned to Debbie and Bob, and though their urge toward contact had not been lessened, the *continuity* of their contact with the baby has been interrupted several times. Here their joy of contact seems evident. Debbie seems relieved and at peace having her baby back with her. Something in the way she is holding the baby gives me the impression that she wants to assert the feeling that THIS BABY IS OURS!

It semed to me that Debbie's joy *had* been a little bit diminished by the separation, but the strong contact, which Bob showed, helped to draw them together as a family unit.

It is important to realize that any emotional interchanges of a deep nature can be very easily interrupted or damaged and even sometimes destroyed by the thoughtless intervention of outsiders. Deep emotional interchanges require a *flow of contact* as they are developing, *any* interference tends to break that flow. The interruptions of outsiders who have no emotional contact with the new parents and have no feeling for them as people is the worst kind of thing that can happen. On the other hand, people who do know, and have good contact with, the parents can *enhance* the growth of these emotional relationships.

It is important to understand the emotional state of the three individuals in the forming family unit. The mother often has been through hours of pain, trauma, and emotionally charged experience and can be easily upset; the baby, whose sensory system is totally vulnerable and wide open, is more susceptible to emotional shock and trauma, probably, than at any other time in its life; the father, of the three family members, has the most undepleted and strongest emotional condition of them all. So it's clear to see how very important and necessary the steady, loyal warmth giving of the father is for both mother and baby during and after the birth.

As Debbie and the baby were being moved from the delivery room to the recovery room, Bob instinctively took a position where he could put his arms around his wife and baby, giving them both all the quiet warmth and

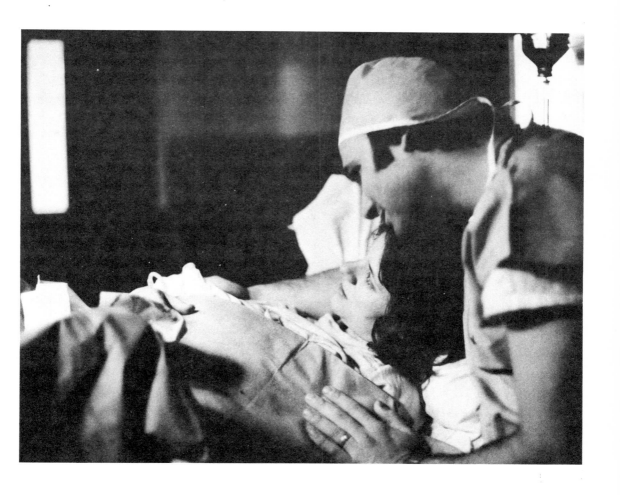

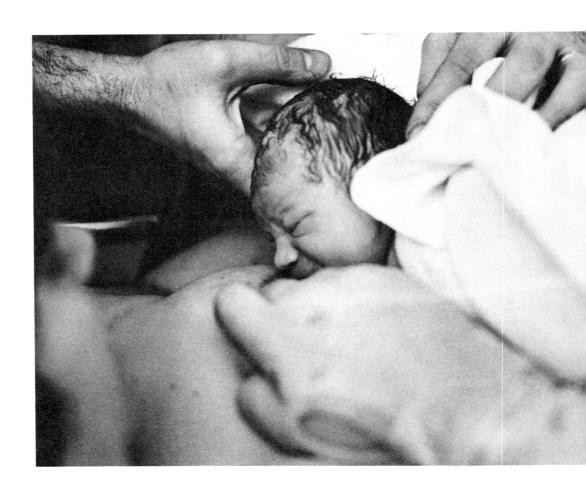

feeling of sheltering that he could. The love that was growing for his new family seemed to flow from him with a very steady and natural combination of masculine strength and gentleness. This kind of male power showed the best qualities that men bring to life. This quality in men is one that doctors, nurses, and hospital directors must learn to understand more clearly and learn to encourage in all maternity situations. But no matter how much encouragement you might want, *you* have to understand one thing: Nobody can really give this strength to you! They can only give you the opportunity to let these things develop.

When it comes time for your own family to be born, there is no telling how many interruptions will occur in the labor or delivery room or how many little traumatic events will happen to your wife and your newborn baby. You might get stuck with having "Nurse Klangbang" working in the delivery room. This is the nurse who has no feeling for the newborn baby's sensitivity, or the feelings of birthing mothers, and least of all for new fathers . . . so you will have to be right there like a great oak tree with deep emotional roots and great, warm sheltering arms. Whatever happens, your gentle touches and looks, your quiet reassurances can hold the whole situation together for your wife and your newborn baby.

Dr. Grover and I visited the recovery room for a few moments with Bob, Debbie, and the new baby girl who had been named Nicole. Here the baby is gently put to her mother's breast, and you see how Bob's hands gently support her head as she begins this very important phase of mother-infant contact.

Though there is no flow of milk at this stage, there is a flow of a substance that is called colostrum that contains elements that are beneficial for the baby and is, so to speak, a forerunner of milk. The nutritive aspects of nursing are obvious, but the nursing process is a most important aspect of emotional interchange between mother and baby. It is a very close reuniting of their two organisms that causes pulsation and flow of feeling between them and excitations within each of their bodies. It is part of the emotional sequence *yearning-contact-satisfaction-deep relaxation* that is identical in many ways to the adult emotional contact and release that Reich described more scientifically as The Orgasm Formula: *tension-charge-discharge-relaxation*. In simpler, everyday language, these things are the feelings of love.

Here in the recovery room, the three family members were to be left alone to give them a chance to draw together. Dr. Grover had been like the Rock of Gibraltar through the whole birth period, doing all that was in his power to enable Debbie, Bob, and their baby to experience the birth in the best way possible. My own admiration and respect for him had grown enormously during the whole experience, particularly when I saw the many difficult factors he had to manage.

So you see, this was not the totally perfect Leboyer-type natural childbirth, and the fact is, there seldom is an absolutely perfect situation in life. But the great and wonderful thing about Dr. Grover is his ability to bring out the best in people despite all kinds of obstacles. For example: He was required by law to see that the silver nitrate ointment was put into the baby's eyes, even though there was no actual need for it with this baby. Despite that, he did everything in his power to prevent that from having any long-lasting effects on the baby through his encouraging contact and a quiet, peaceful atmosphere. Being a highly responsible and dedicated physician, he always works for the best birth possible within the context of the laws and situation in which he works.

OSCAR AND LILLIAN

Radiance and warmth welcomed me when I came into the home of Oscar and Lillian. The kindness and hospitality of these two are remarkable. Lillian is one of the sweetest and most warmhearted persons I have ever known. Naturally, Oscar would have to be a pretty unusual person to rate a woman like her, and he is!

As soon as I walked through their door, I realized that Lillian is not the sort of woman who gives in little bits and pieces and then writes down everything she gives in order to remember it so that she can tell you later; Lillian is a no-holds-barred kind of giving woman. She can't help giving, doesn't want to learn how to stop. She likes making people happy. I fear for her because she has so much guileless generosity. Thank God for Oscar! She'd give away the house if it wasn't for his sensitive restraint.

Oscar is one of nature's wise men. He is also strong of character, intelligent, and a skilled workman. He has these qualities in the same generous proportions that Lillian has her feminine givingness. He radiates a quality of mature, manly capability. One knows automatically that this man can handle any situation that he encounters in life. He is the kind of man who people know can take responsibility in work, and because of this he has shouldered responsibility from a very early age.

Oscar came to the United States at the age of eighteen, not knowing anyone and unable to speak English. He found work in a machine shop. Now, a bit more than ten years later, he is a top machinist who does the highest-tolerance aerospace machinist work. He has been flown all over the country (and to some foreign lands) to work. Having started from scratch on the economic ladder, he now owns several houses and is in the process of buying an apartment building. Oscar is a man who decidedly has it all together.

In this time of antifamily ego aggrandizement, it would be very easy to say that these people are what they are because of their individual strengths. Male and female chauvinists might say that both of these people brought *all* these qualities into the marriage and hold them independently. This was not the case with Lillian and Oscar because, as they have told me, their marriage enabled them to become the sort of people they are. Lillian told me that when the marriage began, she couldn't even boil water; now she is a superb cook and a masterful baker. She learned these things to make life better, just as Oscar learned and developed his abilities for the same purpose.

They met at a dance where Oscar sort of gestured to Lillian to ask her to dance. She wondered why he said nothing to her and halfway through the dance she realized he could not speak English. So she spoke to him in Italian, which was her second language; six months later they were married. They told me that they fought a lot at the beginning of their marriage because they didn't understand one another's needs. Then, they both began to work to make things better and became very close. When you hear Oscar say "my wife," there is a special meaning to the words. Lillian glows when she looks at him.

My evening with them was full of warmth and much laughter. Lillian served the best food imaginable, in great variety and quantity. We talked about the feelings of newborn babies. We talked about how the only way you can let them know that you love them is through soft, gentle touching. We talked about the warmth of loving hands and about how you must hold a newborn baby in your arms with gentle confidence and quiet. We talked about how a baby cannot understand words, but how it can understand the flow of warmth from its mother's and father's hands, arms, and bodies. We three understood each other perfectly.

How good to come to the end of that evening and find that Oscar's very wise reservations about my being with them had vanished. How good it was to feel this good man's warm handshake of friendship. The approval of such a man is worth having!

You can see that Lillian was feeling stress as this picture was being taken, but you can see several other important expressions too. You see a sweet, soft, and yielding love for her husband, a love that is far deeper than any stress she may have been feeling. You see a kindly warm and loving man touching his wife with his eyes as well as his hands. There was nothing forced, nothing held back in the way Oscar cared for Lillian; he was totally self-confident about the warmth that they shared between them. Words cannot really say what their looks and their touch were saying, but it was something as sacred and as beautiful as anything we humans can know in life. I didn't feel like an intruder this time, only a bit hesitant as to whether my presence meant anything to them.

Lillian must have sensed my feeling because right after this she looked at me with her beautiful and gentle eyes and said, "Hello, Nathan," in a way that moved me. Her tone was accepting and welcoming, showing me that she had room in her heart for me as well. I wanted to go over and hug her, put my hand on her brow . . . *do* something because I couldn't help the feelings of wanting to help her. And there seemed to be *nothing* that I could do, though every bit of feeling in me urged me to move toward her. But I stood rooted to the spot and didn't move an inch.

So I went back to the doctors' lounge. I sat there with my camera, ready to go whenever Dr. Grover would call me. I didn't have any of the previous smug feeling of "nobility" about not watching Lillian in labor and "respecting" her privacy; I had an ache, a feeling that I was somehow failing my friends. I felt shut out and helpless because I couldn't help my friends. I wondered over and over to myself "What can I possibly do?" and felt

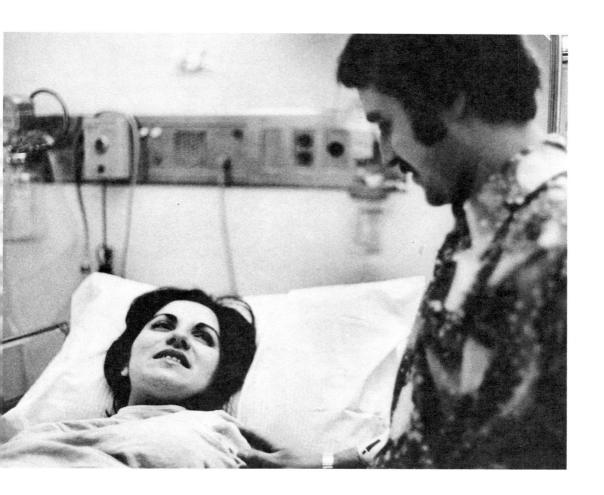

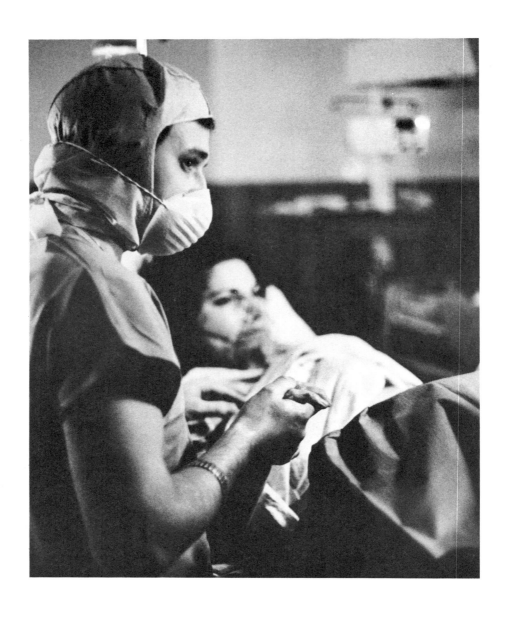

"Maybe I just don't *know* what can be done." "Maybe these are *medical* matters and not my business at all." I felt useless.

Lillian had a difficult and rather long labor. The Lamaze method didn't work in the way it was supposed to and not because of any lack of effort or understanding upon the part of either Lillian or Oscar. I am no expert in these matters, but I later saw several reasons why there may have been difficulty.

One of these may have been the fact that this pregnancy was unexpected, a delightful surprise to both of them and, possibly, something that they felt might not ever happen. I can imagine that Lillian had a very great concern for the baby growing within her and a strong desire *not to lose it*. This feeling may have made her "hold on" a bit longer than necessary.

Another factor that was a worry to Dr. Grover, and was probably a worry to her as well, had to do with a medical condition of a serious nature that Lillian had suffered in the past. It was felt that this condition could have reappeared during the labor. This was another factor that may have made her apprehensive about "letting go."

There was also an unfortunate occurrence that only came to my mind months after the birth of the baby. This was that, through some unusual circumstances, Lillian had to share a labor room with a completely hysterical woman. Having met this woman myself, I can say from experience that her emotional state was enough to unhinge anyone.

At any rate, Lillian's labor was long and somewhat painful, and she finally decided with Dr. Grover's guidance to have epidural anesthesia. With this anesthesia, the woman remains conscious but no longer feels pain and, in addition, the labor contractions are either slowed or stopped. This was the case with Lillian, and her baby did not descend into the birth canal. Because of this, Dr. Grover found it necessary to do a forceps delivery.

When Dr. Grover told me that this would be a forceps delivery, I was very disheartened because this meant that the birth would not be a natural one, but a mechanically assisted one where the baby is actually removed from the womb by forceps that grip the infant by its head. It was anything but a non-violent way of coming into the world to my way of thinking! But there was nothing else that could be done. To my mind at that time, it completely blew any chance for me to observe a beautiful *classical* Leboyer birth. I felt cheated! Yes, I have to confess that my feelings at that time were as selfish and ego-motivated as any feelings I have ever felt: totally small-minded. As it turned out, instead of being a disappointment this birth was one of the major emotional experiences of my life. This birth taught me an unforgettable lesson about the radiating love in Oscar and Lillian. Together in the previous picture they seem to express a simple trust in one another.

I can recall thinking, as I stood there waiting, that the *last* thing in the world I wanted to see was a forceps delivery. On the other hand, I understood that this medical technique *has* saved the lives of millions of mothers and infants in situations where the natural process of birth has been thwarted by the fear-tension-pain syndrome. I knew that Dr. Grover was doing the right thing for Lillian and her baby.

It was absolutely amazing how masterfully John went about the task of forceps delivery. He functioned with swift and economical movements and gave a feeling of confident skill and assurance. More amazing to me was the way Lillian suffered no discomfort. She was bright, alert, and expectant. As all this was taking place, my disappointment reaction changed to a feeling of very deep appreciation and respect for Dr. Grover's abilities. This was still the miracle of birth and there was a very profound feeling within the room.

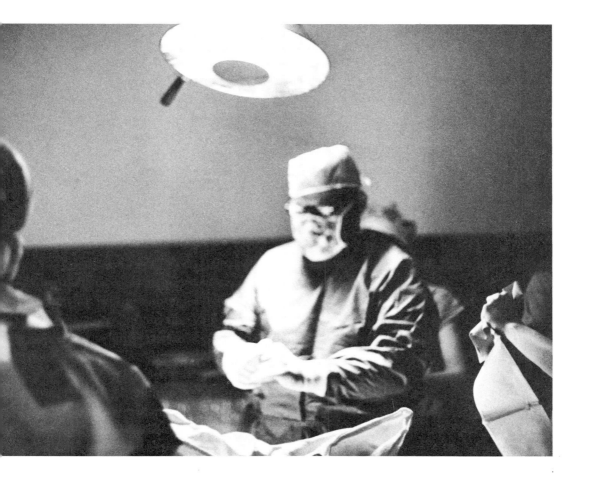

THERE-HERE! With help, yes! With an epidural anesthesia, yes! But it was *right*, regardless; it was just plain beautiful. . . . No. . . . It was *miraculous!*

I think that I saw there in a very short space of time a perfect example of the difference between the imagined ideal and working reality. It was a fine example of Dr. Grover's ability to achieve the best possible results within the framework of his working situation. This baby was met with as much love as any baby born by unassisted means. Lillian was fully conscious, and you can see her eager and loving hands reaching to receive her baby. And Oscar's hands are right there too, just to make sure!

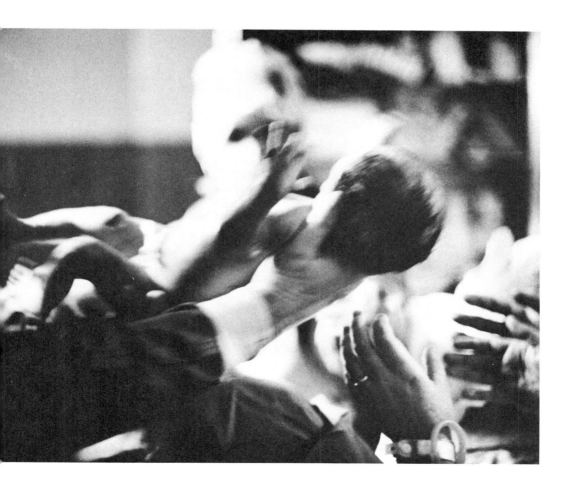

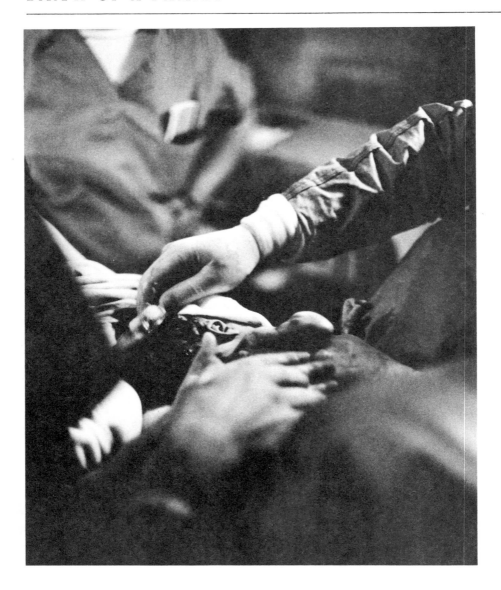

A GIRL! Name? Jamie. As quick as she has been put to rest upon her mother's stomach, both Mother and Father reach to hold her, their hands moving as one.

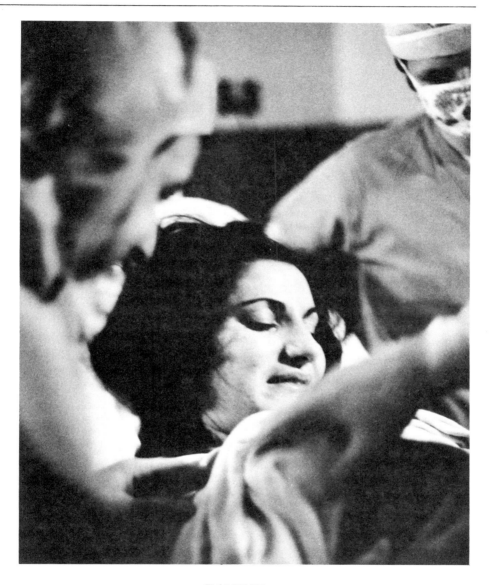

FAMILY!

This soft, gentlehearted woman, her every expression wells up from deep within her soul. Her feeling flows and radiates from her to her baby girl, her husband . . . the world!

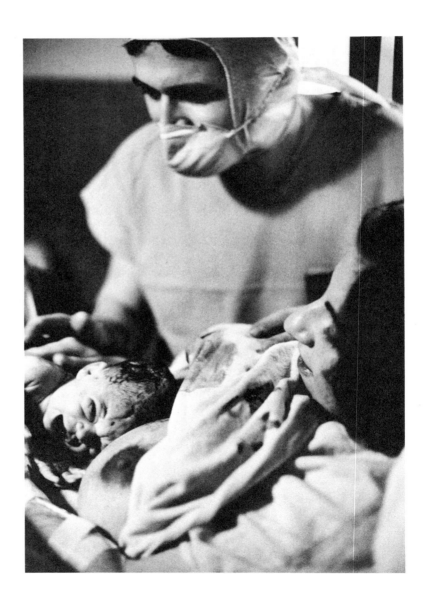

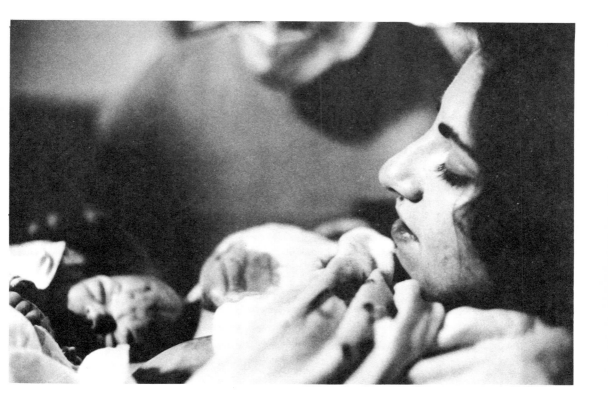

What is the baby feeling? She has had a difficult experience and one can see the marks of the forceps on her head. There is no question that the forceps delivery is traumatic and painful to an infant. It is unnatural and so the baby is expressing hurt, anger, and a certain amount of pure rage. But resting on her mother's stomach, feeling the warmth and loving touch of both the parents' hands is a softening and reassuring experience.

As I looked at the newborn infant and saw those forceps marks on her head and felt her outrage, I wondered how much something like this could

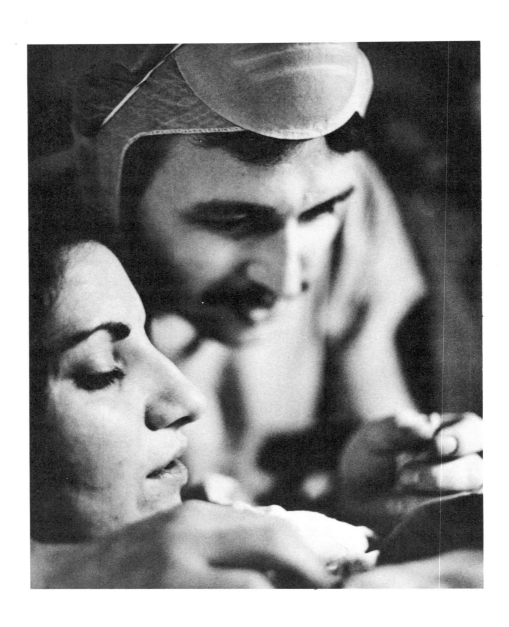

mark a newborn baby's psyche. How many weeks or months would it take for her to recover. The marks would disappear in a few days, but what about the inner marks?

Lillian wasn't thinking any such thoughts; Lillian was feeling delight and . . .

RADIATING LOVE

And Oscar? No holding back of warmth for him! This is probably the best picture that I will ever take. It says everything about a man's feeling for his wife and their newborn baby. Shared delight and closeness . . . these are only words . . . miracle is only a word.

As I watched this take place, I have to admit that grief swept over me again—the loneliness, the feeling of never having had such sweet, shared tenderness. But no jealousy this time. And suddenly, a flood of loving feeling for these two people who are my friends!

Right after I had taken this picture, Lillian turned to me as I stood beside her and said, "Nathan, I just can't tell you what it's like." Because she spoke to me with that gentle sweetness of hers, I knew she *wanted* to share these feelings with me.

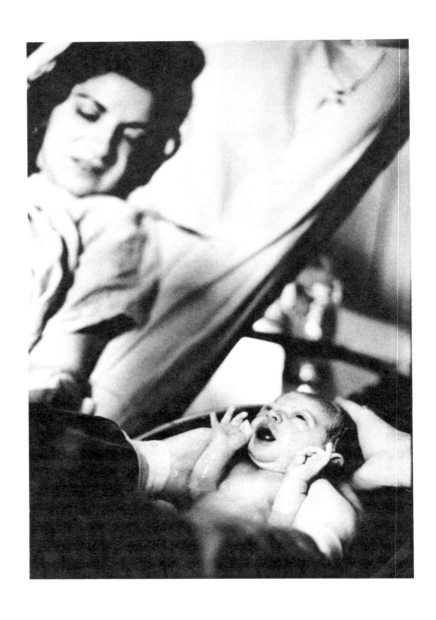

DR. LEBOYER'S MIRACLE

After the umbilicus was cut, the baby was put into the warm bath. As the baby was held gently in the warm water, a major miracle seemed to unfold before me. The crying and rage, which had lessened some as the baby had rested on her mother's stomach, seemed to visibly dissolve before my eyes. Then, her crying ceased altogether and she began to move her arms and legs with beautiful rhythmic movements. She began to make sighing, pleasurable sounds. But what was most surprising of all, the contractions of her eyes, brows, and face disappeared and she began to open her eyes and look around her.

Many medical people who have seen this picture cannot believe that this baby was a forceps delivery, but the miracle was real. The emotional contraction caused by the violence of the forceps removal from the womb was softened by the immediate emotional contact with the mother and father and the resting on her mother's stomach, which was followed by the warm, relaxing, weightless bath. This was Dr. Leboyer's miracle and Dr. Grover's victory.

PLEASURE FOR THE NEWBORN?

Why not? You have to see how much these newborn infants respond to the warm bath to appreciate their unlimited capacity for feeling. This baby seemed to enjoy and feel with her entire body. She felt secure because she was being supported carefully by the hands of Dr. Grover and her father (who never left her for an instant).

YEARNING

For every moment that her baby was away from her, Lillian was linked to her through feeling. But when her baby was taken to the warming table, there was not the sense of broken contact and separateness that Debbie and Bob had experienced because Oscar was there at the table with the baby. And while the nurse was doing the things that were required by the hospital and the state—the identification ritual and the application of the silver nitrate ointment (again medically unnecessary) to the baby's eyes—Oscar never left her side for an instant.

The rage and anger that the baby expressed because of the violence of the forceps delivery, which had so contracted her brow and eyes, was triggered again by the identification ritual and the application of silver nitrate ointment to her sensitive eyes. She yelled and screamed her protest which seemed to be misunderstood and ignored. But Oscar seemed to hear and understand, and every time the nurse left his baby he would gently lay his hands on her body and let his warmth flow from them to the baby. Every time he did this, the baby would quiet down and stop crying. There was one nurse who, whenever she came near the baby, would cause her to howl with dismay! She had that incredible insensitivity to feeling that some obstetrical nurses develop and cover over with a cheery, brisk, self-important bustling that sweeps aside all sensitive feeling. The very presence of the woman seemed to upset the baby, while Oscar's quiet, warm, contactful ways calmed her.

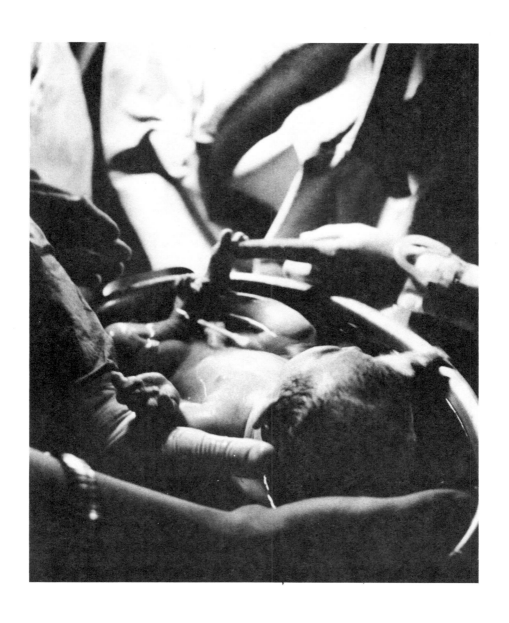

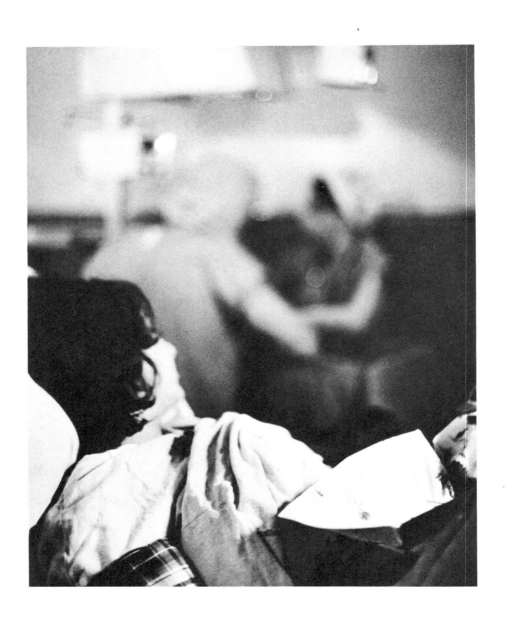

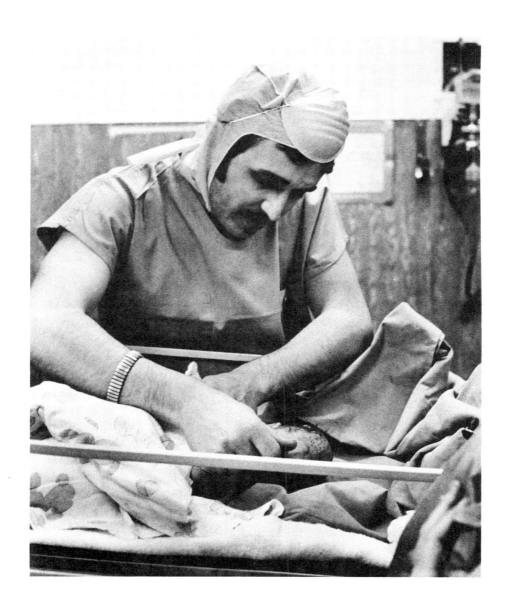

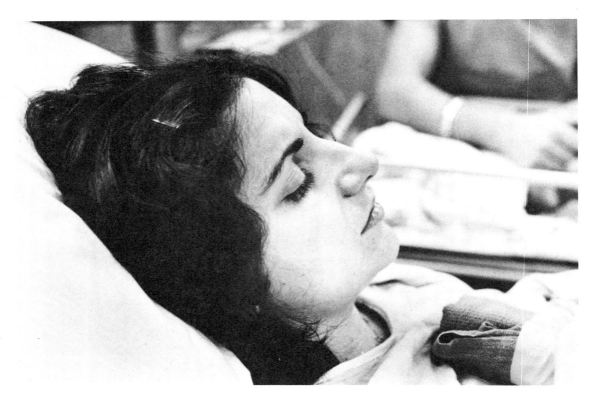

The effect of Oscar's warm and supportive contact with the baby enabled Lillian to sink into a period of deep relaxation. She was able to regain her equilibrium knowing that he was there caring for the baby. She was completely at peace and was able to birth the placenta with ease and not be upset with the stitches that were required to close the episiotomy incision.

There was no doubt that Oscar was completely capable of taking care of his newborn daughter. His self-assurance was very impressive in the quiet and confident way that he managed to be close to the baby at all times. He didn't hang back nor did he appear to push forward in a way that would challenge the nurses; he was just THERE. Something about the way he handled himself gave the sense of authority that this was *his* child and

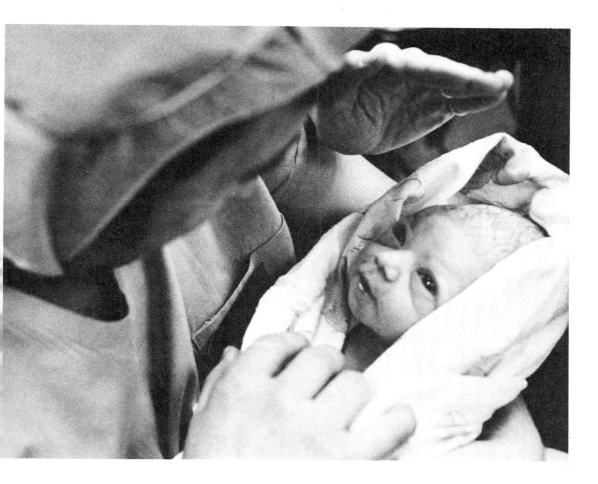

not a property of the hospital, the nurses, or even Dr. Grover. Before the baby was wrapped, he warmed her by keeping his hands gently on her body.

It was astounding to see this little infant try to look into her wonderful father's eyes as if to try (and I'm sure that she was) to express her love for him! She was actually trying to see this warm, beloved person for whom she felt such complete trust . . . HER DADDY!

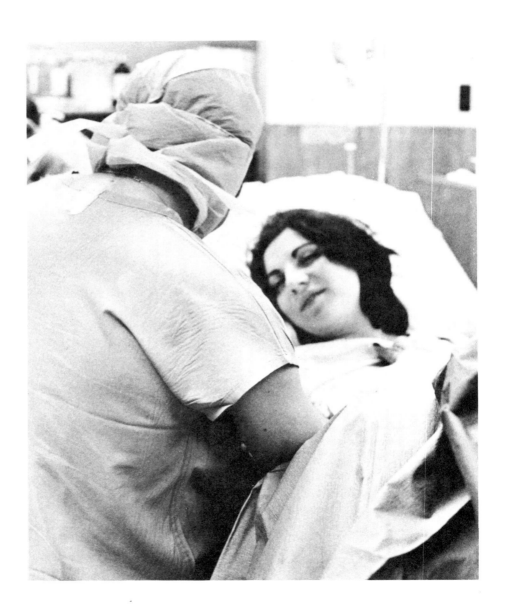

From what had begun with the difficult and discouraging prospect of observing the very kind of delivery that I *did not* want to see, a remarkably beautiful and inspiring experience had taken place. My own ignorance and prejudice had, once again, been shown a truer view of reality. I had learned that what is "natural" in childbirth hinges on many elements and that when one aspect does not operate in the manner one would wish, there are other factors that can compensate and save the day. Lillian's great ability to radiate love and Oscar's warm and steadfast natural instincts as a father flooded their newborn infant with reassuring feeling. And Dr. Grover's judicious management of the whole event and the application of Dr. Leboyer's magic bath had turned what could have been a failure into a glowing success.

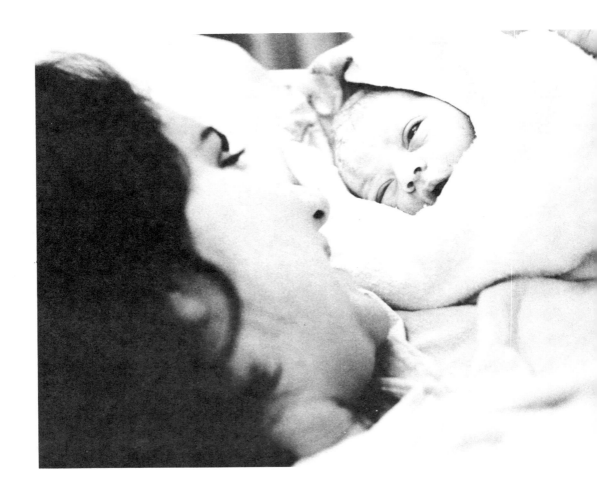

Once the newborn family had settled into the recovery room, the contact of love between Lillian and her baby was easier to maintain. Jamie's little eyes opened, straining through the irritation that had been caused by the silver nitrate ointment, to try to see her beloved mother's face. The great strain and a large part of the contraction of the little face had disappeared, and her expression was that of a delightful and good-natured little person.

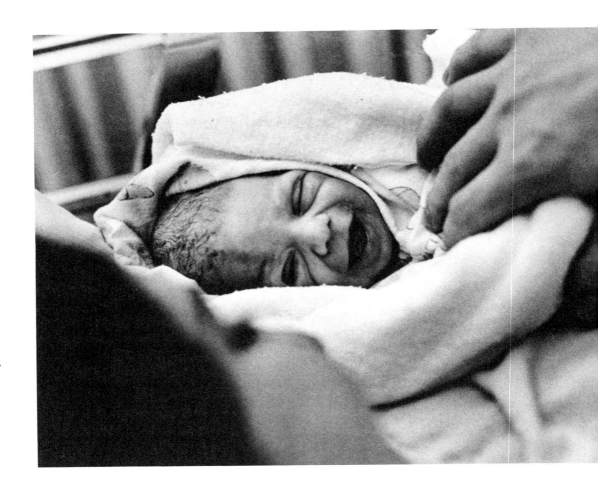

Her father's hand
reaches gently
to touch
his newborn's face.
In responding flood
from the soul's depth
she
releases
the radiance
of her newborn
joy
into
this
world!
for us
to
follow.

I cannot tell you what that moment meant to me. It seemed to be the goal that I had been seeking all the years of my life. In that smile was all the truth, the goodness that I had sought in life. It was the soul's image. That newborn smile has become the cornerstone of my whole existence. It has given me new life. It has given me faith.

Right after this picture was taken, it was time for Dr. Grover and me to allow the newborn family to be together. Before I left, I kissed Lillian on the top of the head and thanked her.

Thanks again, Lillian, Oscar, and you, Jamie, for sharing your miracle with me and with the people who will read this book. Joy to the world!

LARRY AND SUSAN

After I had found my smiling infant, I felt that any further observation of childbirth might be a repetition that would dull the emotional impact of my experience with Oscar, Lillian, and Jamie. I wondered what else I could possibly learn since I had found exactly what I had come to see. But Susan and Larry had something wonderful in store for me.

Of all the couples, Susan and Larry were the ones that I became best acquainted with. I spent more time with them because their baby was born about three weeks after Oscar and Lillian had brought Jamie into the world. In addition, Susan and Larry are about as sociable a couple as one could meet. They are friendly, outgoing, hospitable, full of fun, utterly charming people who are also exceedingly bright.

When I visited them, Susan served a Moussaka so good to the taste and eye that I thought she might be a specialist in Greek cookery. As it turned out, it was the *first* she had ever made! She is that kind of woman—one who gives the feeling that she can do anything she sets her mind to do. She has remarkable amounts of energy. For example: I went for a walk through Boston with her a few days before her baby was born, and she set such a pace that I found it a bit hard to keep up (my excuse being that I am a stroller by nature). "You seem to be a little out of shape, Nathan," was her only comment.

Larry is a man who glows with boundless good nature. He is so warm, engaging, and naturally friendly that one almost overlooks the keenness of his intelligence. He is one of those rare men who has retained the child in himself with no loss to the man. At the same time, there is a very strong sense of self-confidence about him that is not based on putting the other fellow down, but comes from his great fund of warmth and his ability to achieve what he sets out to do.

An important aspect in my relationship with both Susan and Larry was that they were well informed about childbirth, about as aware of the problems involved as it is possible to be because they are both medical doctors. I realize that it might seem unfair to ring in a couple who both have medical degrees. You might feel that you and your wife would be at a disadvantage when compared to a couple of doctors. Though I thought this might be the case at first, the more I thought about it the more I realized that though they might have had more medical knowledge, when it came right down to the labor and birth they had to rely on the exact same knowledge that is available to any parents-to-be who go to childbirth classes.

Susan and Larry had both *seen* childbirth before and had both assisted women in childbirth. But this was *their* first baby and this meant that they had never really experienced birth in a *personal* sense. The factors they had as advantages were *confidence* based on their familiarity with what happens in childbirth, knowledge of hospital procedure, and their own abilities to function in medical situations. This same confidence is something that you and your wife can gain too, as there are limits to the amount of knowledge anyone needs in childbirth. You need just enough knowledge to enable you to reduce fear and to help nature take its course, for it is really nature that does the work.

Susan and Larry were extremely interested in the new approaches to childbirth and the family. They had studied the subjects with great seriousness and were in no doubt about wanting to do the very best for their baby. The baby was wanted, and the pregnancy had been planned so that it would come between Susan's graduation from medical school and the beginning of her residency. She even worked out a special diet supplement for herself while she was pregnant because she wanted her baby to have all the nutritional elements needed for its growth. I had the feeling that these

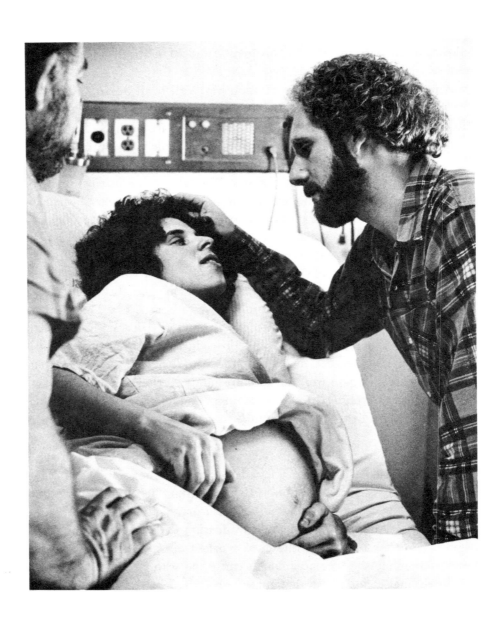

two people enjoyed every aspect of the entire pregnancy, that it was a great adventure for them as well as a great learning process.

Their relationship to me was also very special. Since they had much less anxiety about the pregnancy and childbirth than most people have, they were able to respond to my interests in childbirth in a wholehearted way. They became my teachers in much the same way that Dr. Grover had, and like him, they were interested in my professional insights and gave me the feeling that they might learn from me too. So there developed a four-way mutually respectful association between Susan, Larry, Dr. Grover, and myself that was to lead to an incredibly fine experience for all of us.

There was a fifth party waiting in the wings from whom we all would be learning: the baby. Babies have a lot to teach us no matter who we are; doctors, nurses, parents, observers must learn that it is the baby who does the teaching. All of us must learn to read and respond to the newborn infant's feelings and needs.

When I first came into the labor room in the early stages of Susan's labor, she seemed more confident and "at home" than the other women that I had observed. There were several reasons for this, but the major one was that, as a doctor, she was at the top of the hospital social scale and didn't feel out of place. Another reason for her confidence was that she had been trained to function in hospital surroundings and was aware of hospital routine, personnel relationships, and childbirth processes. All this gave her the sense of being in a familiar place. Larry, of course, had the same kind of ease and confidence that comes from belonging in the hospital environment. Together they had none of the slightly puzzled, out-of-place, and cautious bearing that the previous couples had shown.

This confidence enabled them to move right into their childbirth techniques with ease. It helped them to trust their ability to work together, and it accentuated their highly educated understanding of the physiology of childbirth, enabling them to utilize their trained ability to work as a medical team.

Thinking about this later made me wonder just how much it is possible for ordinary people, who are not trained as doctors and nurses, to ever feel completely at home in hospitals. Hospitals seem to be designed for the convenience of medical personnel in more respects than they are designed to put patients at ease. These thoughts made me understand the reasons why more people are having "home deliveries" and why there are movements afoot to design maternity centers with quarters for patients that have a homelike atmosphere.

As I watched Susan and Larry work together during the contractions that occurred in early stages of her labor, I realized that regardless of their other advantages, the most important thing, underneath everything else, was the close emotional contact they had with one another. It was this that made their use of the breathing techniques effective. This kind of contact is not something that can be taught in childbirth classes so much as it is something that is felt between a man and a woman. This means that doctors can't do this any better than anybody else because it is simply a human, man-woman thing. So this kind of contact is something that you should be able to achieve with your wife if you trust your feelings and open up when you work with her.

I could see that Susan and Larry had put in a good deal of time practicing their childbirth technique, and I imagine that they had felt the practice to be fun rather than a burden. There was no sense of their holding back in any of it.

As I stood watching them, I realized that my own reaction to Susan's labor was quite different from the previous times. Without my even being aware of it, I stayed in the labor room with them for quite some time, watching the process of the contractions with a great deal of interest and no sense of shyness at all!

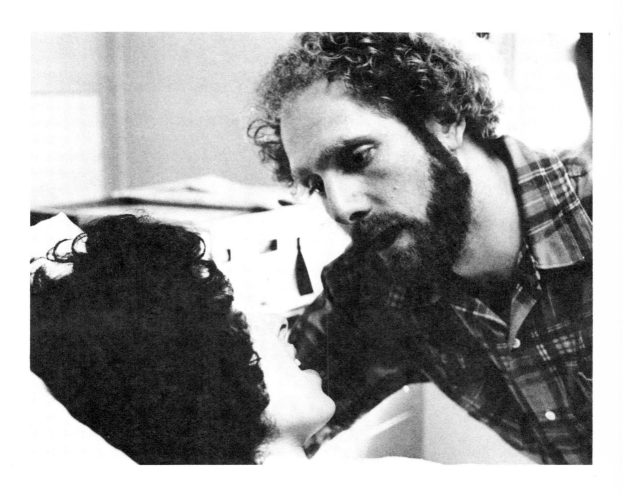

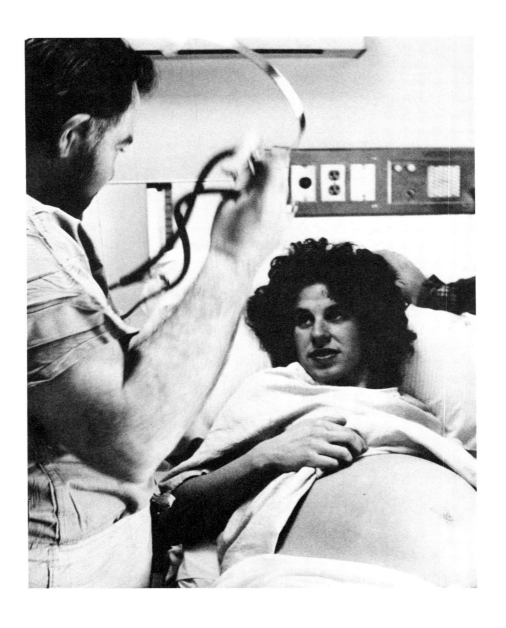

I also noticed that there was a difference in the relationship between Susan and Dr. Grover, compared to the other mothers I had observed. It was easier, and there was a freer communication between them. This was not based on any favoritism on his part, but on the fact that Susan understood all of the factual aspects of childbirth. With Susan, Dr. Grover knew that he was not dealing with a person who only had a vague understanding of the childbirth process. And Susan felt at ease with him because she was able to appreciate the full meaning of all of the things he was telling her about the progress of her labor.

This is something that can be of importance to your own wife as it demonstrates one of the many ways a good, sound knowledge of the childbirth process can help her with the birth of your own baby. Susan knew the facts, so she did not think of Dr. Grover as a superhuman person who knew things beyond an ordinary mortal's understanding. This enabled them to *work together.*

After remaining with Susan and Larry in the labor room for a considerably longer time than I had at the previous births, I began to feel again that I might be intruding, so I went and changed into a scrub suit and took up my post in the doctors' lounge.

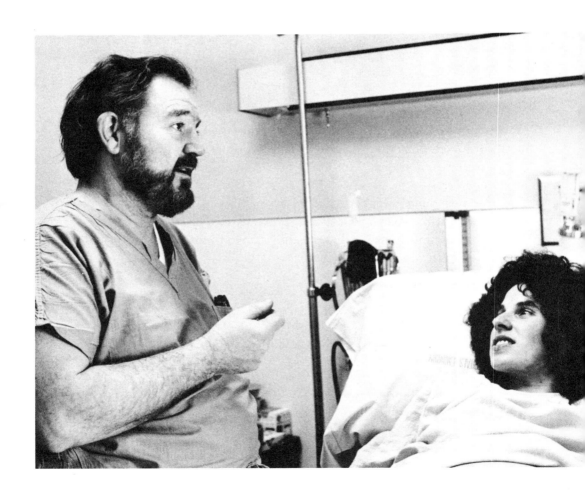

I hadn't been in the doctors' lounge very long before I began to realize that I wasn't where I wanted to be. I wanted to be with Susan, Larry, and John. There had been a different atmosphere in the labor room with them, one that pulled me back against all of my sensitivity about intrusions. I didn't realize what made this attractive force so strong at the time, but months later I saw that it stemmed from Susan's lessened fear about labor, which gave the feeling that everything was under control. I also realized that I felt less out of place with Susan and Larry, and again, months later, I realized that this had to do with the fact that Susan and Larry had a fine insight into the nature of my own work. They respected, valued, and, most of all, *wanted* me to learn from them. In other words I was accepted as an equal, a working member of the team on the basis of *my* knowledge, interests, and needs. So it is not surprising that I soon went back to the labor room "just to see how everything is going."

All of this explains why the atmosphere you see in this picture, during a lull in Susan's contractions, is so easy, good-natured, and convivial.

This photo, taken just a moment later, shows one of the most important factors in this labor situation. This was that Larry was completely at ease about being in the hospital and working with Susan in labor. There was no question about whether he belonged there, no question about his understanding the childbirth process, and also no question about his being able to cope with the situation. And most of all, there was no question about anyone else having to take over his duties.

In this picture you see Susan's complete trust and confidence in her husband. This meant that, because Susan and Larry had learned the facts about childbirth and had learned to work together as a team, the burden of responsibility was not placed on Dr. Grover's shoulders. It made it possible for them to, more or less, take charge of their own childbirth, freeing Dr. Grover so that he could act more as guide and equal participant in the whole experience.

This is the kind of situation that Dr. Grover strives to create in his childbirth practice. By giving over more of the responsibility to the husbands and wives who have learned their childbirth lessons, he enables them to have a deeper and finer experience while he becomes less of an austere authority figure but instead a greater sharer in the miracle of birth.

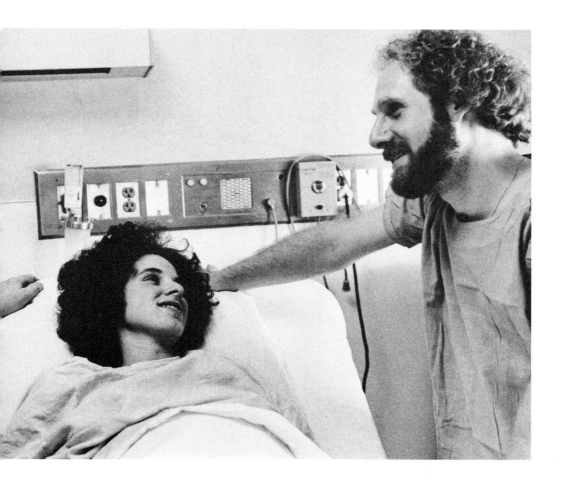

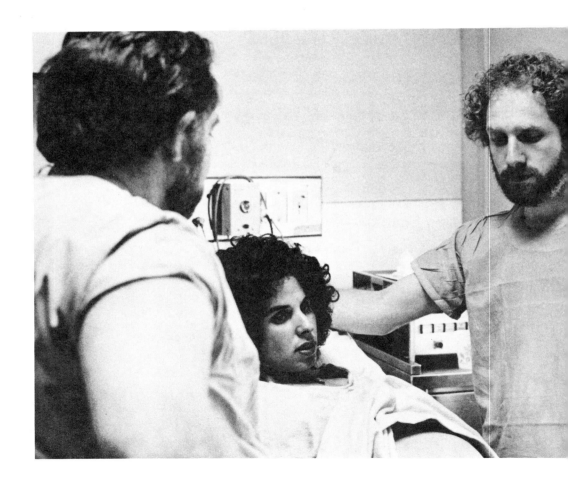

As her labor progressed into the second stage, the mood in the labor room became more serious and everyone's feelings were keyed to Susan's periods of contraction or lull. But despite the deepening of her contractions, Susan remained able to communicate freely with all of the people in the labor room. Her ease in communicating made it easier for them to *respond* to her needs during the contractions. This in turn made for a spirit of good communication during her entire labor, a sense of willing contact. And though I didn't know it at the time, I was later to become a part of this chain of human contact.

Here, Susan was beginning to feel the onset of a contraction while Dr. Grover and Larry were waiting to assist her when the contraction increased in intensity.

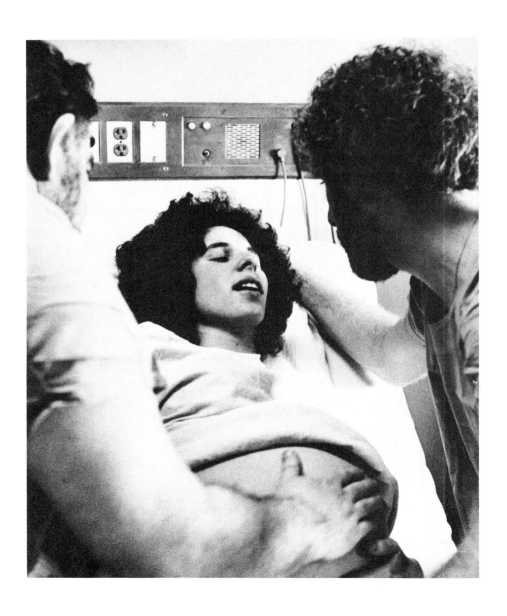

When the contraction intensified, Larry guided Susan into a breathing pattern. At the same time, she and Dr. Grover massaged her lower abdomen to relieve momentary muscular tension to prevent her over-all tension from increasing.

You can see here that during the pain of the childbirth contractions, there is a tendency to close her eyes, break contact, and keep her feelings within. This breaking of contact increases the pain by internalizing it rather than releasing it. Larry was bending toward her here in order to help her maintain visual contact.

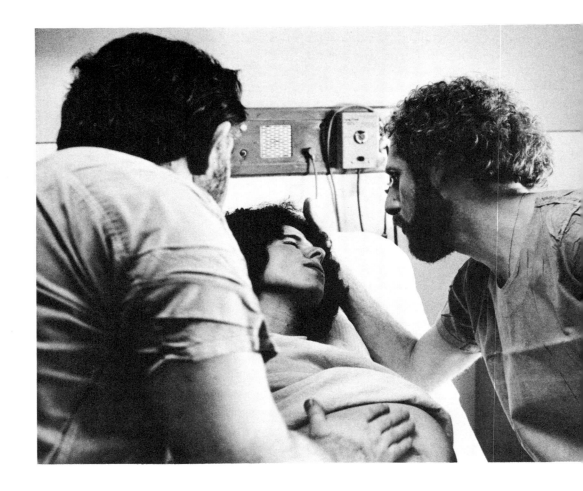

Susan's labor had gone on for some while and the contractions were coming at closer intervals as well as increasing in intensity. Up to this point, she had not had any pain-relieving medication whatsoever and she was determined to do without it completely. This was one of the finest demonstrations of human courage that I have ever seen and it opened my eyes to the physical, emotional and spiritual fortitude many women are capable of achieving in childbirth. But it was something that I could see made a terrific demand on her energy as it became more difficult for her to maintain visual contact due to the mounting pain of the contractions. This demonstrated to me why a woman in labor must have an atmosphere of peace around her and why those who are helping her must be confidently and quietly in touch with her feelings and needs.

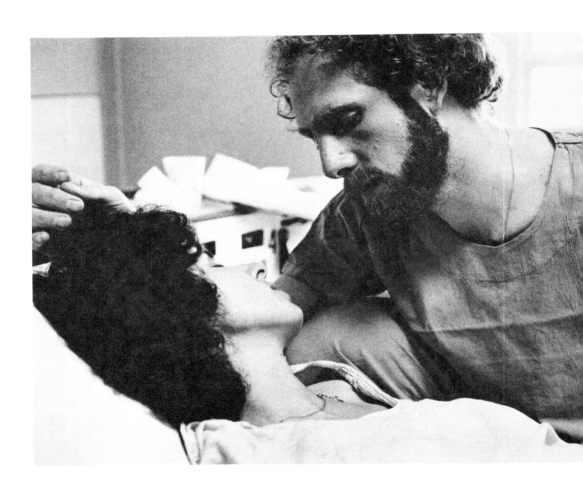

Some time later it appeared to Dr. Grover that Susan was becoming exhausted. He said that her baby was a big one and that this was causing her to expend a great deal of energy moving the baby into the birth canal. Larry was also beginning to show the strain and this made me realize how very strong his contact with Susan was.

Dr. Grover understood from his long experience with labor that Susan needed some rest, but he also understood her desire to have her baby come into the world without having to experience the effect of any drugs, as whatever anesthetic is taken by the mother passes into the baby's system. It had reached a point of crucial decision and I understood why Dr. Grover's guidance was continuously important to both Susan and Larry. He very tactfully suggested that both she and Larry consider the possibility of her taking the lightest-possible medication so that she could recover her strength. This photograph shows the exhaustion they both were feeling at this point.

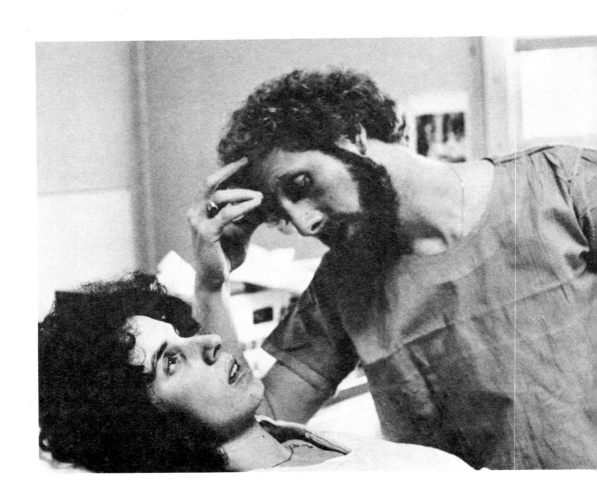

At the moment that this photograph was taken, Susan and Larry had begun to seriously consider the possibility of her taking the medication to remedy her exhaustion. The exhaustion is clearly expressed in her face, but there is also something else, hard to define, that shows she had the will to continue without the medication. I remember her asking Larry at that moment what he felt would be the right thing to do.

This moment showed so clearly how important the role of the father in childbirth can be because this was a decision that they shared between them. Larry knew that Susan would have gone on without medication for the sake of her baby, but he also knew that she was beginning to function on will alone and needed to regain her strength. And because they were so very close at that moment, and her trust in him so great, she knew that she could depend upon his judgment and never have to feel any regret afterward.

"Yes, Sue, you need the rest," Larry said, and it was said with all the tenderness, all the concern for both her and their unborn child that could have possibly been expressed.

Here, two splendid people ponder a question so central to their lives, their sense of personal ethics, and their yearning hopes for their unborn infant. I realized that I was watching a human event of major importance but, strangely, an event that any man and wife in childbirth might experience. If the term "great moments" has any meaning at all, it gains that meaning because every person reaches moments in life that are indeed great and meaningful. It is at these moments that our individual acts count for the whole human race. This was such an occasion, and because of the camera's instant record, we can still observe these two people at one of their bravest and best times.

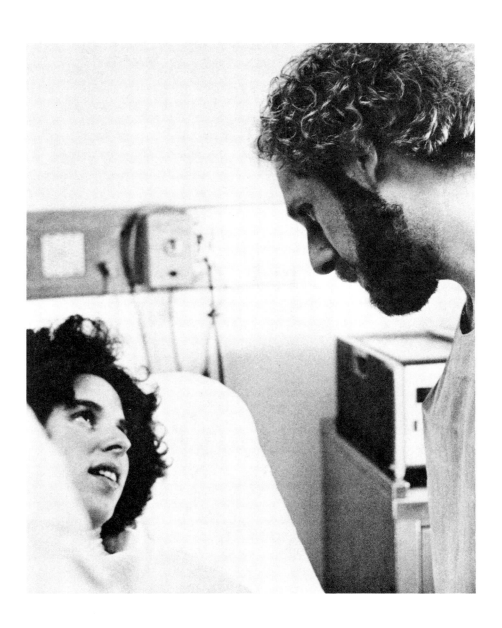

For her depth of needing
and trusting
there was his
visible
commitment of loyalty
and
gentle concern
in
the unconscious
touch of his hand.

*　　*　　*

There was a break in this sequence of pictures of Susan's labor because she was given a very light medication in order to give some relief. At that point, I left the labor room and went back to the doctors' lounge, again thinking to myself that I should stay away from the final stages of her labor "out of courtesy" and wait for Dr. Grover to let me know when she was ready to go into the delivery room. After a little while, something unusual happened and changed everything.

Larry came into the doctors' lounge for some coffee, and he seemed to have recharged his usually boundless energy. He told me how things were going and seemed as vigorous and cheery as could be. As he left to return to Susan he said, "Come on back anytime you want to, Nathan."

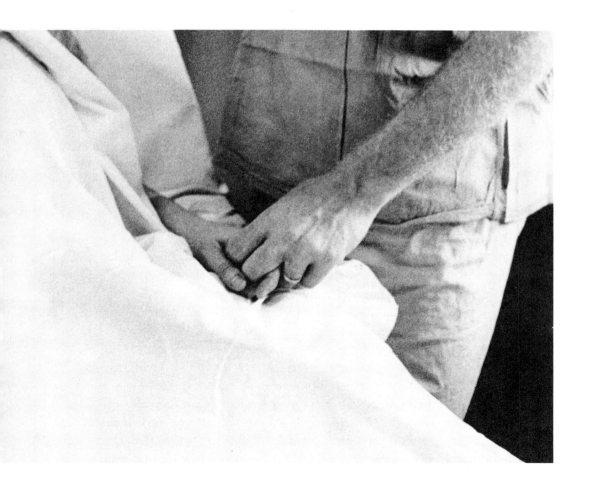

As I sat there for a few minutes listening to some doctors talk of investments, basketball, and other things unrelated to childbirth, I kept thinking of Larry's simple and friendly invitation. All of a sudden, I was on my feet and moving down the corridor toward the labor room. Maybe there was nothing I could do, but Larry had shown me that I was welcome in the most naturally gracious way possible. Maybe just the fact that I loved them would amount to something, and maybe even more important than that was the fact that they were giving me this chance to be with them so that I could learn by sharing their feelings.

When I re-entered the labor room, Susan's contractions were much more powerful and there was a heightened sense of centering in the room. As the contractions occurred, she would call for those around her to help her, and Larry, Dr. Grover, and a young nurse named Lisa would massage her abdomen, arms, and legs to help her stay in contact and ease the tension. It was a tremendously powerful atmosphere to walk into, as she was exerting great energy and concentration. At this time her cervix had dilated and she was working to move her baby into the birth canal.

As I stood watching the rest of them work with her, I felt so isolated that I almost could not bear it. *They* could help her while I couldn't, even though I was powerfully drawn to her every time she asked for help. These calls for help before every contraction were clear and directly honest. "OK, everybody, help me," she would call. It was irresistible; it was a friend calling me for help. All of a sudden I felt ridiculous. Wasn't I one of the world's best natural-born massage practitioners? Didn't I know my anatomy as well, maybe better, than most? Didn't I have my father's warmth of hand? Wasn't I the sculptor of the Cycle of Life?

The next thing I knew I was edging up to the bottom of the bed and rather timidly massaging Susan's right leg, and Lisa, who had been rubbing them both, made way for me. A moment later, Susan in a moment of calm called out: "I wish whoever is rubbing my right leg would put a little pressure into it." That broke down whatever barriers of timidity I had left and from that point on I really went to work with the rest of them. Observing the others, working in harmony with them, following Susan's directions, I became part of the team, a full-fledged member of the birthing of the baby.

The feeling was beautiful, it had a human simplicity. I had never expected it to happen; but when it did, I knew that what I had begun to feel with Debbie, what had grown deeper with Lillian, was as real a human instinct and as deep as any other instinct in life. And what is more, a very natural thing for any man to feel. It was a desire to be involved with something humanly important, something fine and *central* to all life. Then I knew that the birth experience must be the great formative event of human consciousness—the event from which all understanding radiates.

The unity that automatically existed within the group was fine. We were working together for a living purpose which made us close and quietly joyous. There was a keen sense of exhilaration in the room. I felt no more hesitancy and simply did whatever was needed along with the others. At one point, during a lull in Susan's contractions, I even massaged the shoulders of Dr. Grover, Larry, and Lisa and I saw that this touching relaxed us all and brought us even closer together. The smell of birth was like the wind off the sea and it seemed as if the whole human past was with us. I believe that this sense of the biological past must be there with every birth if people will open themselves to feel it.

The final part of the labor remained difficult for Susan as her baby was big and did not turn properly in the birth canal, but by her splendid efforts, the baby began to crown and Dr. Grover eased the lot of us toward the delivery room.

So if you wonder why there are no pictures of the last part of Susan's labor, it was because I was helping my friends. It might not sound like much to you, but it was very important to me, a very good feeling—the feeling of helping with life.

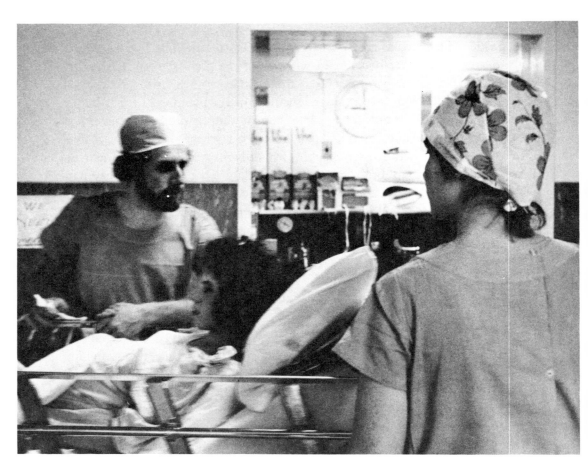

   Now I cannot help but think of the countless women who have been left alone in their labor over the generations and of their husbands who have been denied the simple human right to help and comfort them. No woman should ever have to go through labor alone, without the comfort of a caring husband or compassionate friend. The labor of childbirth is a thing to be shared because it can teach us love and wisdom the way nothing else can.

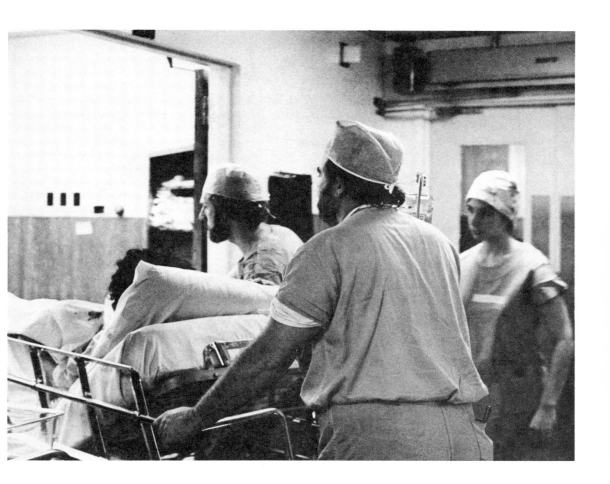

When it came time to move Susan into the delivery room, we all helped to move her bed. Larry seemed to grow in both energy and determination as we moved toward the moment of birth.

Moving into the delivery room, Larry's confidence seemed to expand even more. There was no sense of his holding back or of his shrinking to a

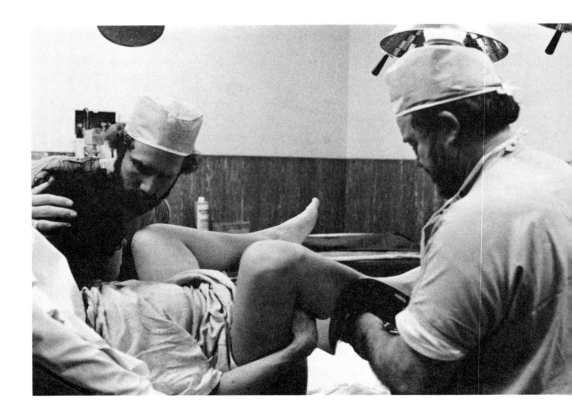

position of secondary importance. All during the labor he had taken a vigorous and leading part and this was exactly what Dr. Grover had wanted. In the delivery room, Dr. Grover tactfully helped Larry to continue his active role and, by so doing, clarified his own function of guiding the whole process and making all of the medical decisions. Of course Larry's medical training was a great help to him in giving him confidence, but it was not essential to the active role he now played under the direction of Dr. Grover.

I know that you might still wonder whether you can ever do any of this as well as a doctor. The point is that *you can* because what Larry was doing was not doctor's work . . . it was father's work. Larry did not do anything during the entire birth process that any intelligent man who had done his homework could not do. Larry being very intelligent *did* do his homework and so he did very well indeed. But what is most important to you, he only did the things Dr. Grover asked him to do, following all directions and suggestions quickly and efficiently.

Dr. Grover and Larry worked well together and quickly got Susan comfortably situated on the delivery table. Larry always followed John's directions quickly and efficiently, but whenever he had completed any chore he simply stood by Susan, giving her his encouragement and tenderness.

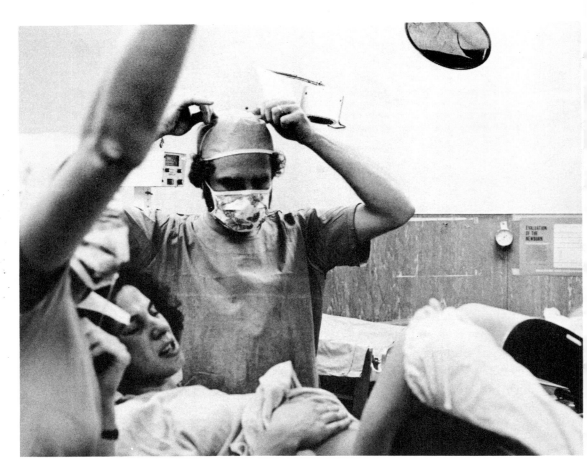

At this point, because of the intensity of her feelings, Susan depended on Larry to keep her in contact. The intensity of emotions and physical feelings right before the birth is incredibly powerful, so powerful that as Larry momentarily left Susan to herself, while he put on his surgical mask, she seemed almost swept away by the feeling.

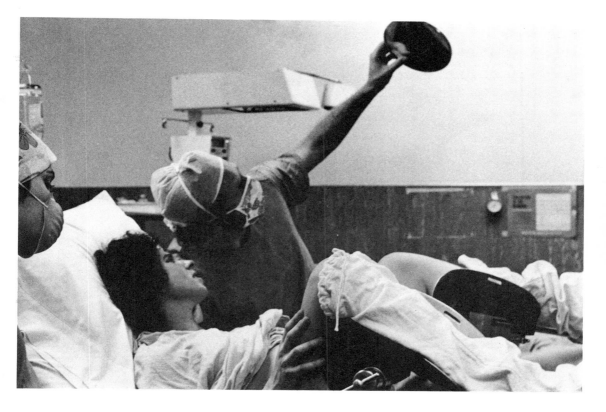

Larry very skillfully worked to keep Susan in contact with him and with the whole birth process. Here, he is adjusting one of the mirrors that enabled her to observe her baby beginning to emerge.

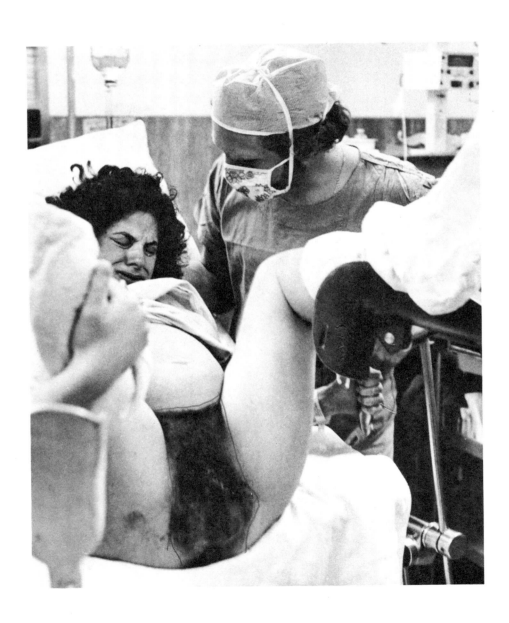

Listen closely to what I have to say. In looking at this photograph, you will have to come to terms with the kind of man you are and the kind of man you want to be. You will have to come to terms with what you think and feel about women, with your stupidities about sexuality, your fears about women, with your understanding of the nature of beauty, and about the very meaning of life itself. Listen closely and try to understand what I am saying because this is important to you.

We men have to begin to understand what women really are and not just what we wish them to be out of ignorance, loneliness, and fantasy. We have to understand what they really are or we will never become what we *could* be unless we can learn about a kind of beauty that is larger than the dreams of boyhood. This picture of Susan can teach you respect for women and reverence for life; it can help you to learn human dignity, decency, and love. Listen to me.

Susan is as beautiful and fine a woman as any woman you will ever know. She is intelligent and capable and as accomplished as any woman you will ever know. She is as loving, as gentle, and devoted a wife as any man could wish for. Listen to me for the sake of your own life and for the life of the children of the future.

What *you* think about women is important. What any man thinks about women is important. Our thoughts are important because they color our own lives and the lives of everyone around us. We men have been little boys for five thousand years and now we must be men. Down through the centuries, we have ridden on the coattails of a few great and courageous men. It is time that we too become worthy of life. It is time that we too learn to revere and protect the life process. The women and the men whose pictures you see in this book have given us visions of their most private moments of birth—for *your* sake as well as mine.

Listen to me.

Now is the time for a new image of life to be born within us.

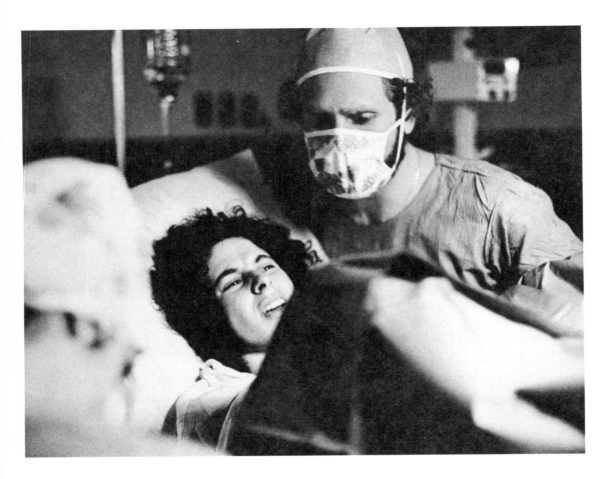

The room was darkened to protect the baby's eyes from the glare of the lights as it began to emerge. With one last effort, which changed from pain to release, Susan brought her baby into the world.

A son, later to be named Joshua, was immediately placed on Susan's stomach to be loved and wondered at. The first thing Susan said was, "Oh,

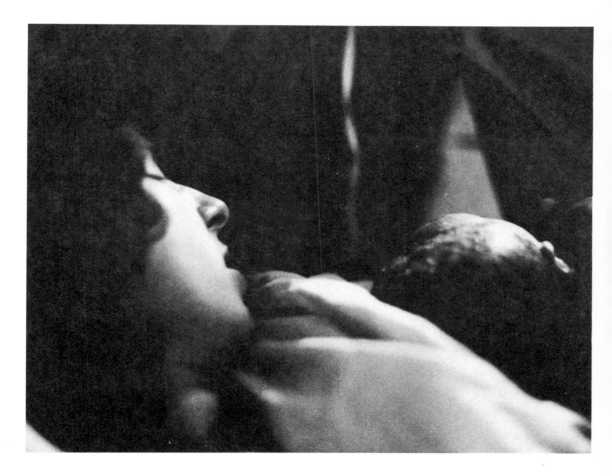

Larry, he's so alert," and it was as though there was no separation at all between the husband and wife. And the baby *was* alert! He seemed to look at
everything around him with a frank and open-eyed curiosity. He showed
no fear; he did not cry, and I was struck by the sense of his *intelligence*, his
alive and open mind.

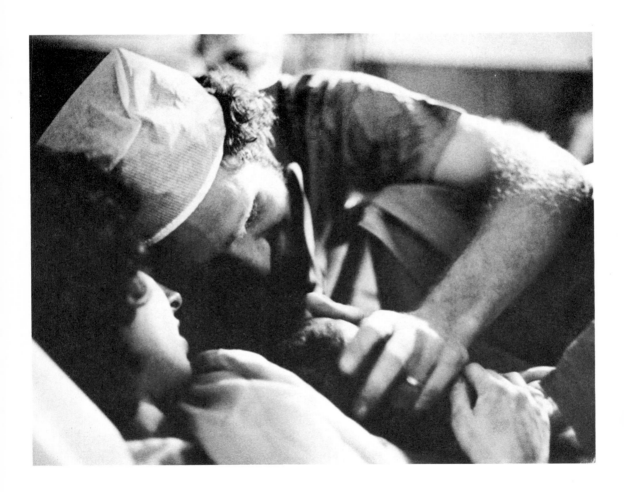

As I stood there watching the three of them, I felt none of the old envy or bitterness because I had been made a sharer of the birth. In my own small way, I had worked for the birth too. Their love was my love and everyone else's and it filled the room with delight.

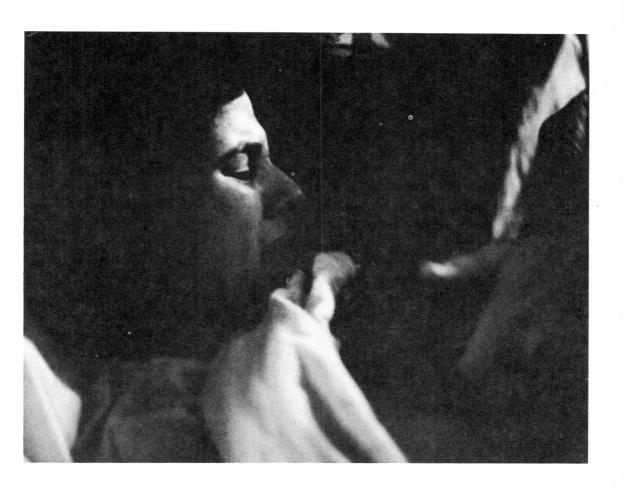

Suddenly, with a sharp cry of panic that shocked us all where we stood, Susan cried out, "Larry, the baby has stopped breathing!" It was utterly shattering to feel the sudden transition from joy to agony in Susan's voice. The room seemed to reel with dismay. Except for John Grover, who instantly spoke in a calm and reassuring voice, telling Larry that he would immediately cut the umbilical cord and take the baby to the warming table. At the same time, he told the nurse to get outside assistance. And Larry recovered instantly from whatever staggering shock he must have felt and began to move with assured and determined calmness.

Nothing could have induced me to lift my camera and photograph Susan in the first few moments after this shock occurred. What you see here is a photograph taken after she had heard that her baby had begun to breathe again. The depth and range of emotion that had crossed her face had been enough to tear my heart out. For a few brief moments, I had shared with her the feeling of shock and utter helplessness. Some of this you can see in the expression of her eyes and the gesture of her hand as she began to recover.

The baby was in perfectly fine health after having what Dr. Grover called a laryngal spasm from a bit of mucous that had lodged in his throat.

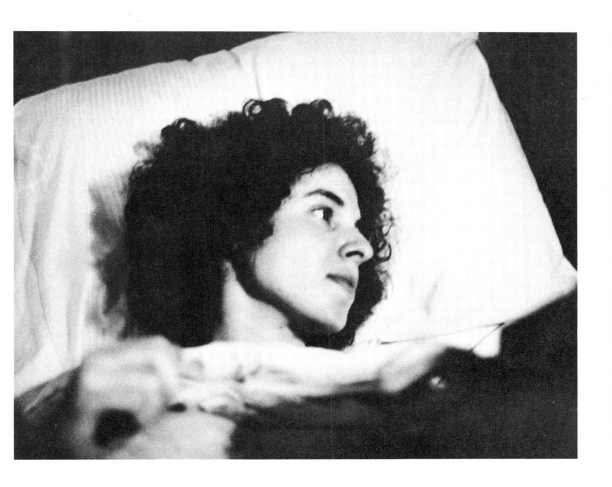

Not only was the baby all right, he appeared to be a remarkably well-formed baby. His look of intelligence and bright-eyed curiosity were startling. No one could have seen that baby and maintained any of the old belief that babies don't possess all of the human feelings and awareness.

Babies who have been anesthetized may have that groggy, half-conscious look, but this baby showed why Susan had fought so hard to resist taking any medication. She had wanted her baby to come into the world with all his feelings and emotions open so that the birth of his *consciousness* would be unclouded.

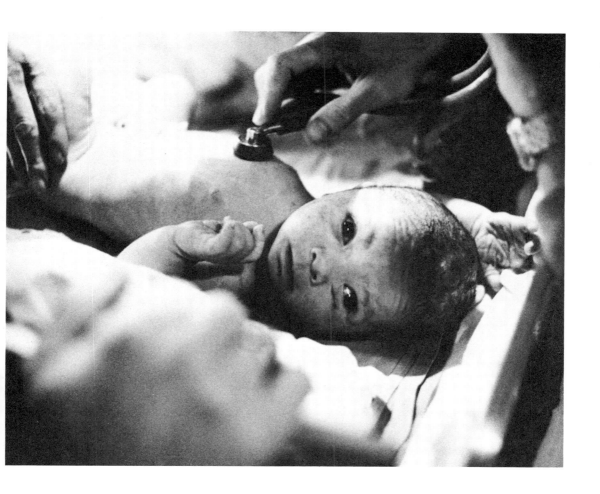

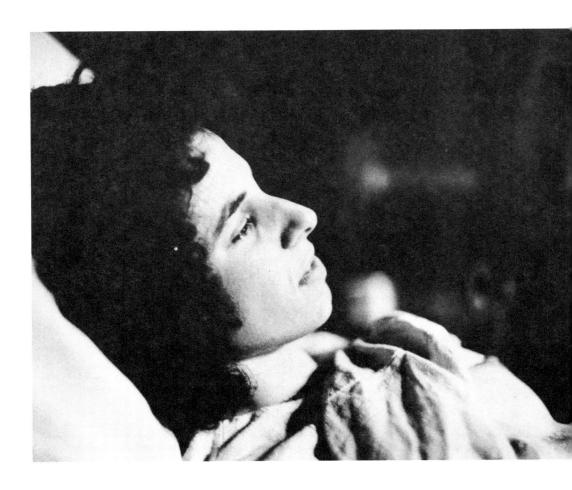

Susan's recovery was complete in a matter of a few minutes, and it was a lesson to me of the astounding resilience of the human spirit. It was also helped considerably by Dr. Grover's cool handling of a potentially devastating situation. Larry, too, had no small part in the emergency treatment of the baby. When Dr. Grover said everything was all right, Susan believed it. But when Larry said everything was all right, she *knew* it was so; the tension left her and she began to recover her energy. Surprisingly, recovery seemed almost instantaneous. Her general lack of fear, her knowledge of the childbirth process helped to keep the shocks and contractions she had experienced from depleting her energy. At the same time, her confidence enabled her to feel everything intensely during the whole birth experience.

In the meantime, Joshua began to show some annoyance at the noise, the strange hands, and the separation from his mother, so Dr. Grover suggested that it was time to put him into Dr. Leboyer's soothing bath.

The expression of this newborn infant was direct and forceful. I could see why some people are actually frightened of the feelings of infants. There was tremendous power and energy in this baby's expression of feeling; it seemed to come from the very core of his life . . . direct and true. By the same token, the change of his expression back to calmness was clearly noticeable, when he had settled into the warmth of the bath.

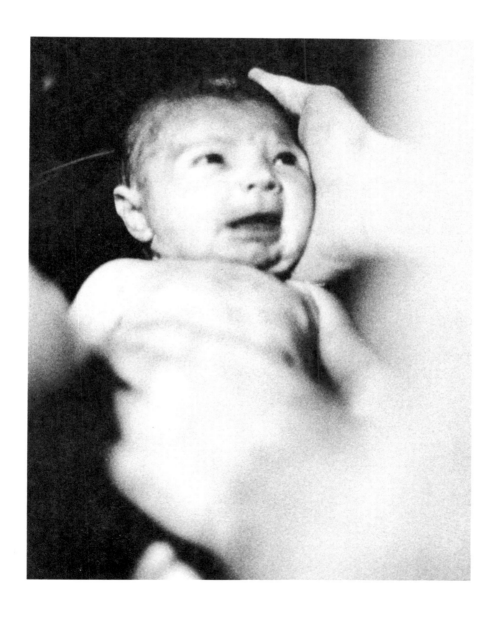

Larry was with his son during all this time, giving him his warmth and strong emotional contact. He felt no hestitation about holding his baby and sheltering him with the warmth of his arms and hands.

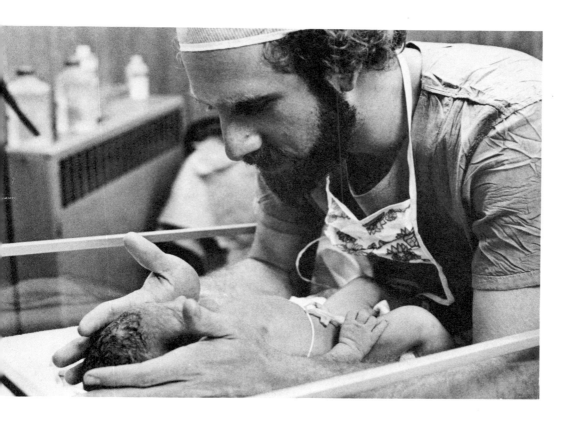

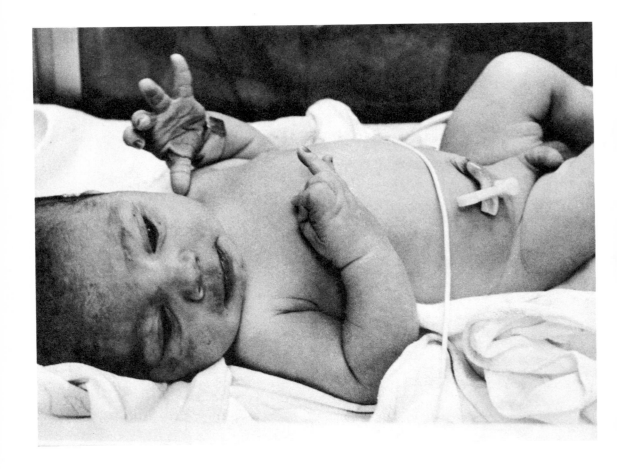

After the soothing bath, the baby was taken to the warming table for the identification routine and the treatment of the eyes. But this time, instead of silver nitrate ointment, the baby was given an antibiotic salve that had no irritating effect. Both Susan and Larry knew about the effects of silver nitrate on the sensitive eyes of newborns and had specially asked that the antibiotic be used instead.

You can see that there was no contraction of pain in this baby's forehead, brow, or eyes, none of the puffed-up painful look that had been caused by the use of the silver nitrate ointment in the other newborns. So instead of having to make a painful effort to see what the newly entered world was like, this baby was able to look with open curiosity.

Many people who have seen this picture find it hard to believe that this is a newborn infant, because his body wasn't contracted and because he was so relaxed and in contact with his surroundings. The simple fact was that he had not been drugged by anesthesia, had not been pulled into the world violently or been held by his heels and slapped, had not had his eyes shocked by the glare of harsh lights and later had them burned with irritating medication. As a result, there was no armored contraction of his body musculature, and he had every reason to be absolutely delighted with life.

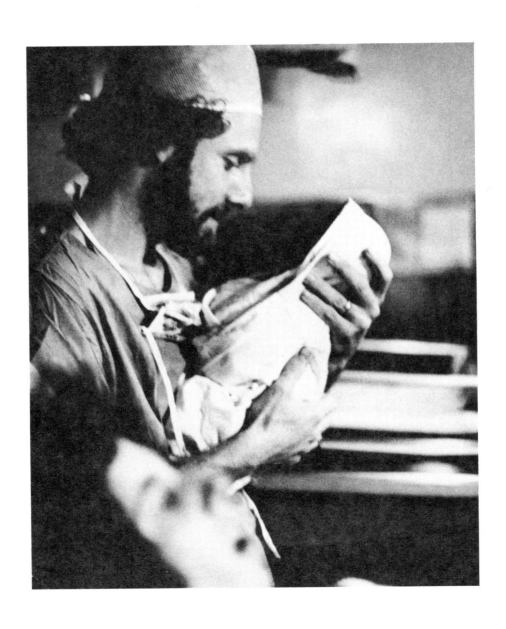

Here you see a father who has *reason* to feel pride in his newborn son. This father has *worked* to bring his son into the world in a gentle way and, from the very beginning, has done his best to protect him from harm and the unfeeling treatment of strangers.

And there is no doubt that the newborn child is finding out who the gentle and protective man may be. . . . that familiar presence.

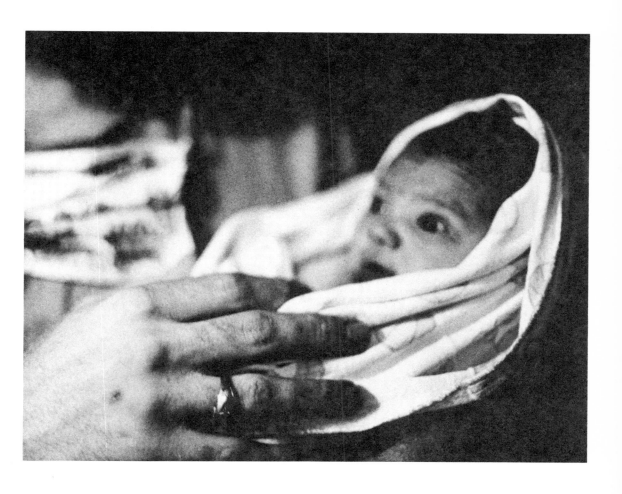

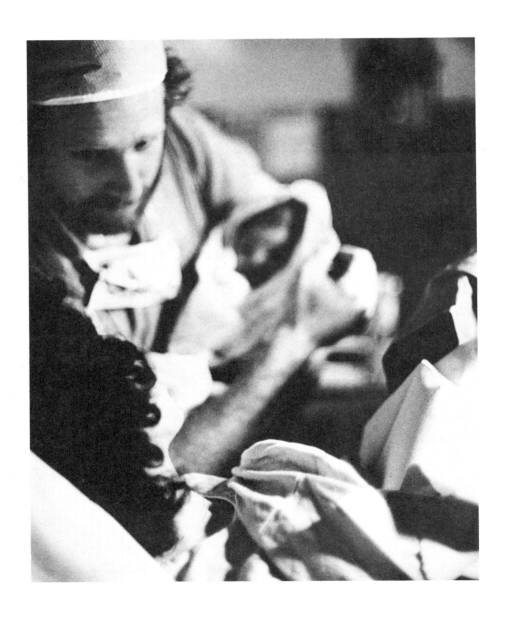

As Susan was receiving final medical attention from Dr. Grover, Larry held the baby for her to see, but I believe that it was not only the baby that she saw. I believe that she saw that she had given her husband joy; I believe she saw his newly minted fatherhood; I believe she saw *her family*.

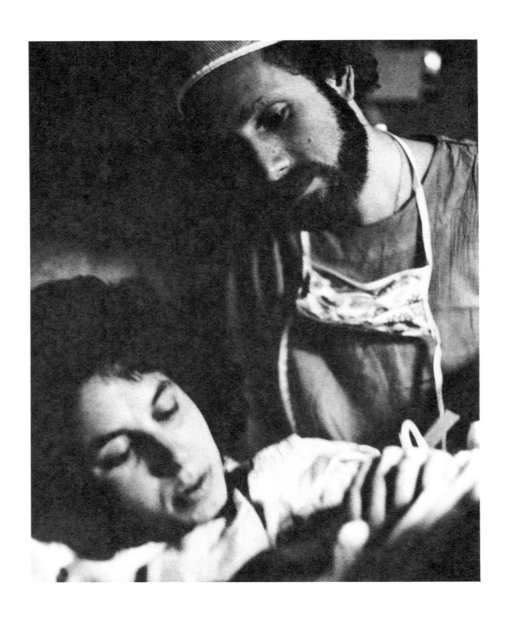

Woman
is everything . . .
our world,
our universe,
that for which
we reach
and yearn.
In finding
her
she gives us
rest.

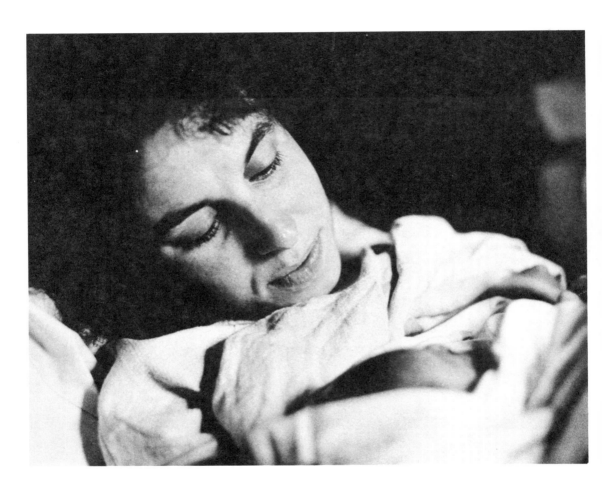

Turn back for a moment to the picture of Susan in labor (see page 154). That picture was taken only a few minutes before this one. I want you to understand that the gentle sweetness and adoring love she shows to her newborn infant here has a certain price. Understand that we cannot ask women to carry the whole burden of life alone. Let's make an agreement here and now between ourselves, a simple agreement to work for, and with, life. If we can begin to do this, we will begin to understand woman's beauty and maybe even help it to grow.

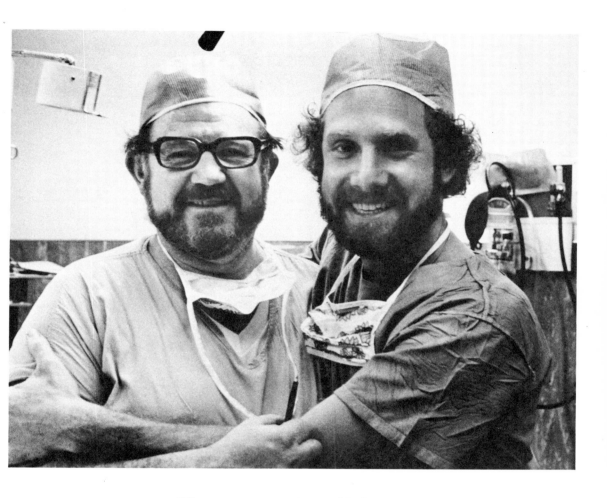

That man to man, the world o'er,
Shall brothers be for a' that.
Robert Burns

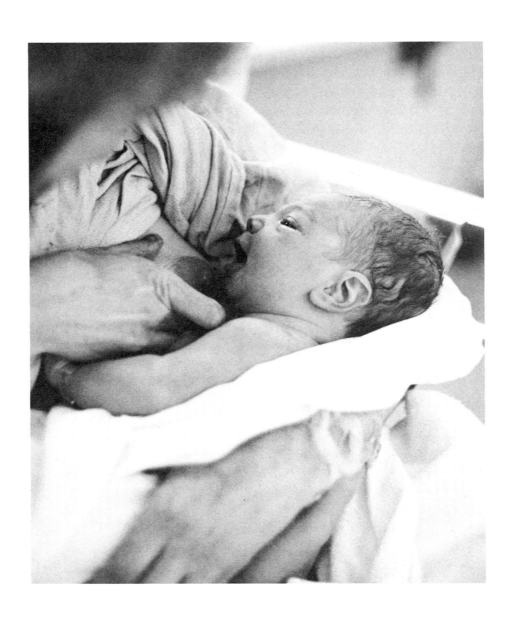

This photograph was taken right after Susan, Larry, and Joshua entered the recovery room. And though I am not quite sure whether Joshua was smiling or not, he seemed to be in high good humor and ready for his mother's breast.

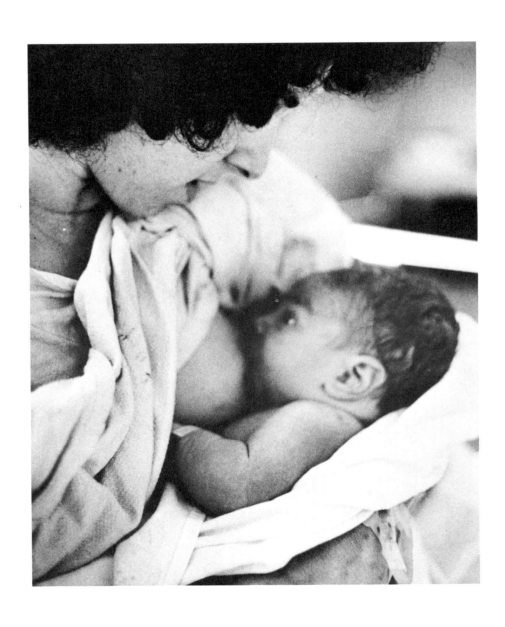

As soon as Joshua was put to the breast, it was clear that his sucking reflex was strong and unimpaired. Susan commented with delight, "He sure knows what he's doing." And this was another reason why she had wanted to avoid any anesthesia, because it has been found that anesthesia has the effect on newborns of inhibiting their ability to nurse.

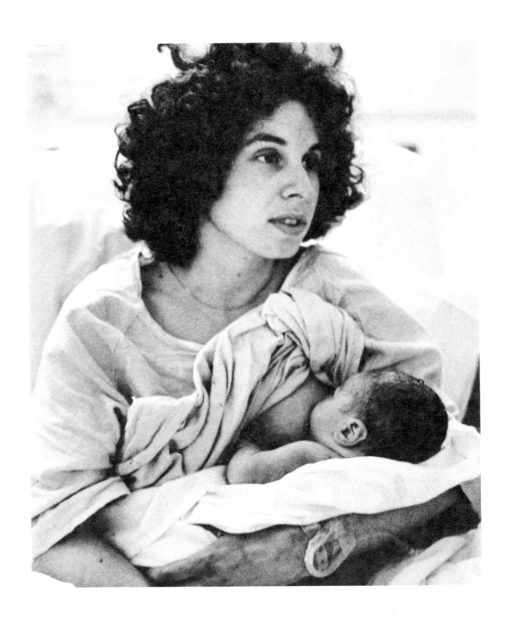

Though she was new to motherhood, Susan showed no awkwardness or hesitation; her every move was easy and natural and a marvel of instinctive competence. It was hard for me to believe that I had seen this same woman going through hours of emotional intensity such a short time before. I am not sure that men can really ever fully understand women, but we have to try; and even if we do not ever completely understand them, we *can* marvel at their mystery and love them more dearly for it.

As John and I were leaving, Larry hugged Susan. Then she kissed him tenderly and simply said, "Thank you, Larry."

*   *   *

With that gentle comment, Dr. John Grover and I left them. As the two of us walked down the corridor, I felt the glow of comradeship between us, the kind of feeling that can come to men when they work together and the work goes well.

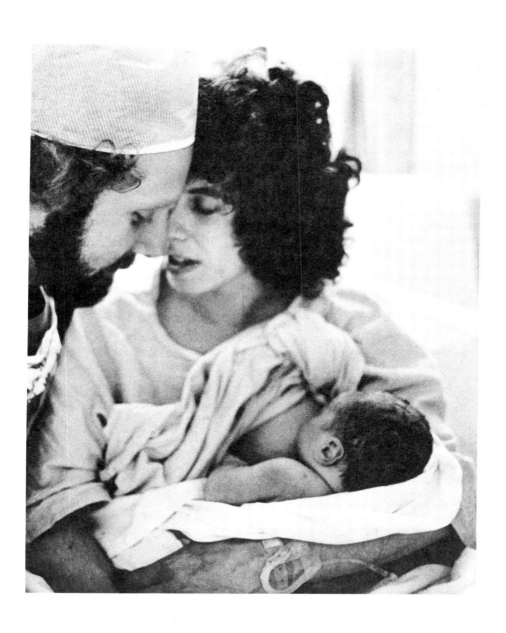

A CONCLUDING DISCUSSION

Now that you have shared these birth experiences with me, I think that you will be able to see how great a role feeling and emotion play in the experience of childbirth. I think that you will begin to understand how important it is to protect and encourage these feelings and emotions during the birth of your family. I believe that perceptive and sensitive men will understand these feelings from looking at the pictures. However, all perceptive and sensitive men will find it hard to understand why the kind of birth we have shown here *is not* the way birth has been managed in the past and is not the way birth is managed in the world today, in the majority of cases. The dominant approach to childbirth is still a much more impersonal and mechanized one.

This mechanized approach to childbirth is based on the application of *sterile surgical technique* and mechanical understanding of the birth process to actual labor and delivery. In this approach there is a blindness to the emotional nature of the human infant. In addition, the mechanical approach does not take into account the natural feelings and emotional needs of the mother. But the most excluded and least appreciated is the father, who, in the mechanical approach to childbirth, is the forgotten soul and not seen to have any function at all in the birth process. The mechanical approach to childbirth has grown so far away from human emotional reality as to seem actually monstrous in the light of what natural, non-violent childbirth so clearly reveals to us. I will enumerate both approaches in order that you may judge for yourself the truth of that I have said.

The Mechanical Approach to the Childbirth Process

1. *Exclusion of the father* from labor and delivery and denying him any natural role in the childbirth process that can improve conditions for his wife and newborn infant and show that he has a deep emotional and developmental need to participate.

2. *Mechanical hospital environment* with tile walls, machines of unknown purpose, surgical instruments and knives, routinized and impersonal treatment by mechanically efficient and emotionally indifferent strangers.

3. *Labor in fear and loneliness* where the woman in labor often hears the agony and frightened cries of other women, which augment her own fears as she has had no preparation for labor or instruction in the techniques of aiding the natural process of birth.

4. *Anesthesia and stupefying drugs* routinely given which blank out the entire experience of birth and also hinder the natural contractions and expansions of the labor process, making emotional contact with the newborn infant impossible.

5. *Episiotomy incision* is routinely given (the incision is a large one for the following activity and convenience of the physician).

6. *Forceps delivery* routinely applied to the infant, the forceps being clamped on the infant's head for the purpose of pulling the infant from the womb.

7. *A drugged and semiconscious infant* as a result of the medication and anesthesia given to the mother, which has passed automatically into the bloodstream of the infant. This impairs the infant's ability to respond to the necessities of birth with clear reflexes and clear emerging consciousness.

8. *Violent treatment of the infant*, making violence its first conscious experience. After being pulled from the warm and sheltering organism of its mother by a metal instrument clamped to its head, the newborn is held upside down by its ankles. This stretches and pulls the musculature of its legs, spinal column, and neck—which have grown in soft repose in gentle

curves—into a violent and terrifying weight-bearing extension. This is immediately followed by a sharp slap on the buttocks, which is supposedly given to "start respiration."

9. *Immediate separation of infant from mother.* The just born infant is held by strangers, the umbilicus severed (often before it has stopped pulsating), and the child is taken across the delivery room to the warming table.

10. *An immediate series of traumas to the infant's eyes* occurs at birth. First, the glare of the harsh surgical spotlights; next, by application of the stinging silver nitrate ointment; and, finally, through the attempts to make contact with the indifferent and loveless eyes of strangers.

11. *Isolation of the just born infant from all loving contact.* The infant is then put through the identification process, labeled and wrapped, and taken to the hospital nursery by a totally unrelated and uninvolved stranger.

12. *Prolonged separation and deprivation of maternal and paternal contact.* The newborn infant is kept in the hospital nursery with other infants, who have been similarly treated and who are frequently screaming in desperation, for periods that range from twelve to twenty-four hours (and sometimes longer), during which time contact is denied to both parents. In addition, the infants are *not* held for purposes of contact by anyone during this time.

13. *Circumcision* is routinely done by the mechanistic physician, when he can obtain the consent of the parents (and he always urges them to consent), within the first few days of a male infant's life. In this surgical operation, the foreskin of the newborn infant's penis is held by metal forceps while this protective shield of sensitive flesh is cut away from the exquisitely sensitive head of the penis . . . without anesthesia! The penis is the most sensitive external male organ, the most subject to emotions of terror and to permanent psychological trauma.

The effect of the mechanical approach to the childbirth process is the production of a series of violently contracting, emotionally damaging traumatic experiences that are routinely applied to newborn infants at the period of their greatest openness and vulnerability. This approach completely eliminates all warm, contactful, and loving experience during childbirth for the infant, the mother, and the father. This approach to childbirth reduces it to a series of mechanically performed steps that obliterate the central, emotionally formative experience of family life.

In long-range terms, it is hard to assess what this kind of emotionally devastating and unnatural distortion of the birth process will produce (or has already produced) in this culture. One thing is certain: The elimination of human feeling from the primary human formative experience can do much toward turning humans into armored beings more akin to *machines that feel* than to warm, compassionate, and loving men and women.

I hope that you will now be able to understand my deep concern about the mechanistic trends of thought I observed at my Harvard lecture and why I feel that this kind of mechanical thinking is a threat to our own everyday lives, to the lives of our children, and to the future of life on this earth. But what *you* do in the formation of your own new family is more crucial to the future than the words or theories of any scientist (be he right or wrong). Your family *is* the future and that is why it is important for you to take responsibility for whatever tasks of childbirth you can fulfill, with the help of your wife and your doctor. The more you study and work with your wife, the better the two of you will be able to create the finest kind of childbirth experience.

The Natural and Non-Violent Approach to Childbirth

1. *Participation of the father,* wherever possible, throughout labor and delivery. This is based on the degree of desire for participation, the amount of knowledge of childbirth gained, and the ability of the husband to work with his wife as part of a team.

2. *Homelike environment* in the hospital, or an actual home delivery, ensures the sense of comfort, peace, and relaxation in the mother so that she can experience the natural rhythm of her labor contractions and expansions.

3. *Labor in peace, without fear and without loneliness.* Because the husband and wife have both learned about the process of labor, they are able to work together to prevent fear and loss of contact mounting to create undue pain. The experience of labor becomes a shared experience in which the man is able to *give* something from his own heart to help his wife in giving birth.

4. *No anesthesia or drugs* are forced upon the mother who wishes to remain conscious and in contact with the whole childbirth experience. But medication is available to her whenever she feels she might need it.

5. *No episiotomy required* in cases where good relaxation is achieved and the the mother is able to give in fully to the contractions and expansions of the labor process. In other situations, a smaller episiotomy is required than in the mechanical approach to childbirth.

6. *Natural delivery*—the infant emerging through the natural expulsive process of the contractions and expansions of the uterus and womb.

7. *A conscious and responsive infant,* not stupefied by drugs and anesthesia, is able to enter the world and experience the birth of its own consciousness and loving contact with its own parents.

8. *Gentle and tender treatment of the infant* rather than violent handling and harsh slaps. Awareness of the infant as totally open in its feelings and perceptions, a creature of complete vulnerability, possessing *all* the human feelings.

9. *Immediate contact with the mother.* At the instant of birth the infant is placed on its mother's stomach to rest, the umbilicus is not cut until its pulsation stops, and its breathing is allowed to begin spontaneously.

10. *Immediate relaxation of traumatic muscular tensions* with the use of the warm Leboyer bath. This allows the infant to once again achieve the warmth and weightlessness that existed for it in its mother's womb and to

relax any of the tensions that may have occurred during its struggle to achieve birth during the period of labor.

11. *No traumatic assault to the eyes of the newborn,* first because the room has been darkened down to a functional, not glaring, light, with the turning off of the surgical spotlights. *And most important of all,* the infant's eyes have not been shocked by the application of the stinging silver nitrate ointment. No medication is given unless needed, in which case a non-irritating antibiotic ointment is used. It is recognized that since the eyes are such a direct extension of, and in such close proximity to, the brain, a trauma to the eyes at birth is the most shocking type of mental birth trauma possible.

12. *No separation from maternal and paternal contact* and no emotional deprivation produced by isolation. The infant and parents are never separated, as they go right to the recovery room together. It is then kept in the room with the mother (in the rooming-in hospitals). And of course in home deliveries the infant is "at home" and among his or her family from the very beginning. The infant is allowed to nurse within a few minutes after birth.

13. *No circumcision of the male infant* because it is understood that the penis is a sensory organ of the most vital importance to life. It is understood to be a sensory organ of both perception and response, the function of the foreskin being to protect the sensitivity of the head of the penis, which is the area of greatest perception and response. The preserving of this sensitivity is vital to the future life of the male infant because as a man he will perceive and respond to his beloved with whatever capacity his sensory system may possess; the deeper his responses and feelings, the deeper will be the union. The greater his sensitivity and the greater his perception of the beloved woman's feelings and changes, and the greater will be the radiations of responding warmth, pulsation, and sensitive movement. To perform this operation on a newborn infant results in traumatic shock as well as a lifelong coarsening of the deepest sensitivities.

The effect of non-violent natural childbirth is to reduce the number of shocks and possible traumatic experiences for the newborn infant. But non-violent natural childbirth does not stop there; it also employs the Leboyer bath and warm and tender physical contact to counteract whatever accidental shocks may have occurred in the course of the labor and birth. The warm and loving contact with the parents, the avoidance of contact with unfeeling strangers, and the warm and weightless effects of the bath not only dissolve muscular tensions, but also create an atmosphere of quiet joy. The whole approach allows the natural progression of the emotionally ful-fulling events that bring about the birth of a family.

So, non-violent natural childbirth fosters the experience of life's most important formative event for the infant, the mother, and the father. It allows the infant's consciousness to be born in a quiet atmosphere of love and wonder. It allows the mother to experience the birth of her child and also the birth of her husband's entry into fatherhood. It gives a man the opportunity to affirm his wife's courage and to help it grow. It gives him the opportunity to demonstrate his loyalty and devotion to his wife and new-born infant. And perhaps most important of all for the man, it initiates him into the great mystery of woman's awesome creative link with the great designer of the universe. And to *anyone* who shares this experience, it makes possible the great step toward the feeling of "reverence for life."

A Final Note

As I told you earlier, I had to leave Boston before the birth of Eric and Laura's daughter, Jessica. But I did return, with Dr. Grover, to visit them the day following the birth of their baby.

They told me that everything had gone well and that they had missed me. I was glad to see from the happiness they expressed that what they missed wasn't something they lacked, but rather that they had missed being able to share their happiness with me.

Dr. Grover had told me that Eric had done a first-rate job of helping Laura with her labor and had excelled during the delivery too. I had known that he would and was delighted to see the effect this had on their newborn family. When either one of them spoke of the baby, there was always the feeling of *our* rather than *mine*.

Being with them again made me happy in another way because it was a *return*, and I had been a bit sad to leave Boston and the close friends I had made there. But the thing that pleased me most was something Eric said as Dr. Grover and I were leaving. He said, "I almost forgot to tell you, Nathan. Right after Jessica was born . . . she smiled."

As you'll recall I did not begin this project with the idea of writing a book, but the simple and direct words of this good man told me that there was no book around that spoke to fathers.

I have always believed that good men don't need much explanation; they see and feel what's right to do and then go ahead and do it.

My wish is for your strength, your loyalty, your devotion, your tenderness, and your courage. With these, you will find the love of woman, the newborn infant's smile, and the touch of the great designer of the universe.

RECOMMENDED BOOKS

From my own point of view, the following three books are the finest on the subject of childbirth.:

DICK-READ, GRANTLY, M.D., *Childbirth Without Fear*. New York, Harper & Row, 1970.

This is the best all-around book on labor and childbirth. It will probably never be surpassed because it was written by the founder of the natural childbirth movement.

LEBOYER, FREDERICK, M.D., *Birth Without Violence*. London, England, William Collins, 1978.

This is the best book about the feelings of childbirth from the viewpoint of the infant. It fully describes Dr. Leboyer's great contributions to the technique of childbirth.

BAKER, ELSWORTH F., M.D., *Man in the Trap*. New York, Avon Books, 1974.

This book was written by a leading psychiatric authority on muscular armoring, the effect of shock and trauma on the human psyche. There are sections on prenatal care, the nature of babies, and infant care. There is also information on the negative effects of circumcision.

1994